managing *your* image

laurel herman

Published by Positive Presence

ISBN 1-905493-03-7

Originally published by Hodder & Stoughton for the Chartered Management Institute.

Printed by Athenaeum Press, Gateshead

contents

First and foremost, this book just has to be dedicated to my long-suffering family and all the team at Positive Presence who support me so well.

It is then also for our loyal clients who have contributed to my experience and expertise over the years. It was their support, appreciation, increased confidence and achievements that helped me to realise the significance of image optimisation. In reality, it is just the converse of "spin". It should not create false illusions, but strongly and irrevocably convey all that is positive about you so that others appreciate you for the person you are – your attributes, achievements and your abilities.

Laurel Herman November 2009

preface

Over the last few years, Positive Presence has developed basic image consultancy to a groundbreaking level, **Impact Optimisation.** Entitled 'YOU are your own best Business Card', the programme is delivered to groups as training, 'motivating' or 'edu-tainment' and to individuals in the form of coaching or enhancement. *(see back pages)*

As it is YOU, when YOU walk in the door, who win – or lose – the job, the deal, the relationship .... or whatever else is at stake, the importance of the first impression cannot be overstated. By helping men and women maximise their Impact and Presence, they raise their profile, enhance their career prospects, initiate and develop relationships and get listened to, taken seriously, respected and remembered positively. They then are able to get more from people, situations... and life.

Impact optimisation focuses on every aspect of how you sound, look and behave. As others perceptions of you will be based on each of these, but judged collectively, they must be authentic, (i.e. true to you), congruent, appropriate .... and optimised in order for you to be judged as a Positive Presence.

This book was originally written for the Chartered Institute of Management to a specified brief regarding Positive Image. It therefore does not cover each of the impact aspects in equal detail and, although it has since been updated and self-published, it still maintains its original focus and format. I am therefore adding a few paragraphs about Impact to supplement the information that follows in the book.

Your own level of personal Impact is a decision instantly made by others at their first encounter with you. If their perception of you is positive, and/or if they recognise that knowing you will be to their advantage, they will want to meet you – and to get to know you.....and then to get to know you better too. It is then up to you to do your utmost to develop the relationship.

Few services or products are unique. If they are, they are soon emulated. Business today is about people and at the end of the day, people buy people rather than organisations. So, if you are seriously seeking to enhance your career or your business, it is paramount to first acknowledge the importance of people and their relationships with you.

Your relationships with the people you already know are most important and should be strengthened and personalised wherever possible. But you also need to grow the number of people you can call contacts, if not friends, in order to increase your visibility, raise your own profile and create opportunities for development. The easiest way to do so this is to build a network.

NETWORKING

Much is heard and being written about networking today and to many, the principles being advocated (or the lack of them!), feel uncomfortable, insincere and in opposition to their underlying beliefs and values. The Positive Presence philosophy and proposition is entirely different; it is based on your personal integrity, authenticity and sincerity. It helps you to appropriately identify and develop opportunities, develop your own profile and appropriately interact and communicate dynamically in all situations.

Networking is the easiest way to expand beyond those you know already. But the way you do this must feel 'right' for you, comfortable and attainable. Meaningful relationships first have to be initiated and then only over time can be built on firm foundations of mutual trust, empathy and rapport. Of course you need to consider who else could be good for you to know to further your business or career. However, the Positive Presence golden rule is that your networking should absolutely not be confined to finding and developing those who you believe could do so. By displaying respect to all you encounter, showing (and feeling) genuine interest and being generous of yourself with them, you will undoubtedly benefit in some way from most people over time. To make others feel valued and liked is critical but to do so you must maintain regular contact, however time-poor you are and difficult this may be. It can never, ever bode well to contact someone only when you patently have a need or are trying to sell them something – or yourself.

INITIATING RELATIONSHIPS

To build your network, you have to meet people face-to-face even if the initial contact may be by email, letter or phone. Consider attending any group activities run by professional bodies, membership organisations, SIGs or charities that would appear appropriate to the type of person you would like to get to know. You will then begin to expand your own network base which will grow exponentially as you become more adept at social-business networking. Remember that each of your new found contacts will have their own web of contacts which may also be an important fund of potential new ones for you too. But don't appear predatory; first allow your contact to build trust and confidence in you before suggesting a referral.

Some people find the concept of 'working the room' formidable, even dread the idea of initiating contact with one other. It is far better to begin or develop a relationship with two or three significant people than attempt to make a number of new contacts for the sake of it. Quality not quantity! All the advice given in the book about getting your image right now applies because others will instantly make numerous significant judgments about you when they first meet you. Your level of impact and presence to them is critical to your hopes for building a future relationship.

Whether in a meeting or at an event, most relationships start with small talk (however else?), find some level of empathy, build rapport and then move into significant, more meaningful conversation. This can certainly be helped along by giving away a small nugget of considered and appropriate personal info which help them to get to know you better too. You, and they, are people, not merely job titles. As time goes on, you can offer a listening ear, contacts, social opportunities, information, support, guidance, companionship – in fact, whatever else that is needed, but only if it is appropriate at that stage of your relationship.

Personal networking is one of the most effective ways to promote yourself and get more out of life as well as progressing your career or business. But constantly remind yourself that good networking is a two-way exercise – and giving most definitely comes first and foremost. The gain *may* come later. Networking and relationship skills can be learnt and mastered once the need to do so is recognised and accepted.

IMPROVING EXISTING RELATIONSHIPS

Of course, at Positive Presence our work is not only about securing new relationships by maximising the First Impression, but focuses equally on analysing and improving existing ones too. There are always some people we cannot seem to get the best from, some with whom we are just not comfortable and some with whom we do not have the type of relationship we should – and could. Dealing with these specific situations is out of the scope of this book but relationships can usually be improved by identifying why and how others react to us and then utilising the information to make some appropriate adjustments to our communication and behaviour.

There is a very successful device we often use to turn around negative judgments that have been made by significant others at the first encounter. Because we are all living in a very visual world, appearance is very, very important in all first impressions that are not by phone or email. By adjusting your appearance, and for the better, you will find that people are provoked subconsciously into revisiting their first opinion of you. So if you have changed over time, and are since communicating and behaving in a more positive way, they may well be induced to see you in a new and improved light by making some tweaks here and there to your appearance. And even if they don't, your confidence will increase because the 'Look Good; Feel Good' factor kicks in!

The aim of **Managing your Image** is to make you more aware of the importance of your image, dispel any misconceptions around this subject (so much rubbish is written!), motivate you to make some adjustments and then to give you some basic tools to make your image a more positive one. Then, by adding your enhanced image to good networking and relationship building, you will begin to accrue the many benefits, both personal and professional.

May your good work begin…

Read on!

Laurel Herman November 2009

an introduction to managing *your* image

Your image is how the world sees you. Obviously this matters most when people don't really know you or about your abilities, qualities, achievements etc. However, even when they do know you well, they still retain their own original image of you based very much on what they thought when they first met you. Psychological research proves conclusively that the First Impression is very powerful and many decisions are made instantly. Those judgements collectively create a filter through which you and your behaviour are seen from then on and the original decisions are rarely re-visited, let alone changed. In other words, the viewer's perception of you is believed by them to be the **reality**.

Because of that importance, you should do your best to ensure that the image others have of you is the one you would want. That is what managing your image is all about. To do it successfully, we need to examine how that image is created initially and then the ways in which it can be adjusted if it is necessary.

You need to be aware of the significance of your image to you and your career and we shall explore the way that you can use it to your best advantage. Image is a composite of all that is seen and heard and we will identify and examine the various Image Ingredients of which it is made up.

Before we start the 'improvement, enhancement and development', you need to stop and think hard about what you would like your image to be. It is then both useful and enlightening to test how others currently perceive you. This will help to determine your strengths and weaknesses and create our strategy.

We will continue by working through the Image Ingredients one by one and you can apply the advice when you think you need it.

Having dealt with all the different aspects of how you are perceived, you should then feel confident that you are truly managing your image – and most positively. As your confidence increases even more, as it undoubtedly will, your overall image will become more positive too.

Old habits die hard and as life takes its normal course with the usual stresses and strains, it is really easy to slip back into old ways. We therefore must also find ways to help you maintain the enhancement, check that it is being sustained – and deal with any sudden crises.

By the end of the book, you will have a truly positive business image that will most certainly be viewed more positively by others.

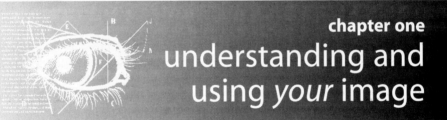

understanding and using *your* image

Your image is

OTHERS

perception of

YOU

In Britain we sometimes have a problem with the word Image, but far less now than used to be. Many people used to believe that if they were judged by their image, their quality of person, let alone their ability and intelligence, were being compromised. But today, helped by Reality TV, makeover programmes and the emphasis on personal development, this is now changing.

> Whether you want it – or not,

> Whether you like it – or not,

> Whether you agree with it – or not,

There is no doubt that to everyone you meet for the first time...

> Initially, you are an image.

However, the good news is that *you* are in control of *your* own image.

It stands to reason therefore that you should create, or adjust, it and use it to the best advantage in both your personal and business life.

Overall, the **right** business image is one that says you are:

Flexible	Approachable	Competent
Confident	Energised	Experienced
Honest	Intelligent	Organised
Professional	Resourceful	Reliable
Sincere	Successful	Communicative
Efficient	... and on the cutting edge	

the importance of *your* **image...**
... as a tool of **communication**

The modern world is all about communication. It is also an essentially visual one due to the universal influence of the screen, both large and small.

When an advertising agency or a film director wants to create a character that you will recognise instantly, they will portray a stereotypical image that leaves you in no doubt.

Similarly, **you** too can be a stereotype that is easily understood by others and gain instant credibility. Should being a stereotype feel uncomfortable, let me add that you are able to adjust it to 'your own' version. On the other hand, if you are so obviously **not** the stereotype that people recognise instantly, you would be taking a risk in that you may well not appear credible at first and therefore will have to prove yourself so much harder.

the first impression

Much has been written about the First Impression and I do not believe that anyone today can deny its importance. We all admit to making instantaneous judgements about others; it is therefore obvious that others make them about us too.

However, it is interesting to discover just how many *subconscious* assessments we make, either **rightly or wrongly.** When you meet a business contact for the first time, there are many decisions you make about them instantly without ever realising it. For example you definitely decide about their gender, age and ethnicity – but there are also at least 20 more. Enter below any that you can think of on Table 1.

table 1		
judgements		

Of course, it must be true that when others meet you, they equally make similar decisions about you.

In reality, these will include a selection from:

Authority	*Ability*	*Energy level*
Aptitude: sporty, creative, etc.	*Background*	*Career potential*
Cleanliness	*Confidence*	*Corporate commitment*
Determination	*Dynamism*	*Education*
Flair	*Lifestyle*	*Health & wellbeing*
Honesty	*Intelligence*	*Regional origin*
Marital/family status	*Meticulousness*	*Orderliness*
Personality	*Poise*	*Political orientation*
Class	*Sense of humour*	*Sincerity*
Social attitude	*Status*	*Wealth*

In business, when your image is in any way perceived negatively by the respondent, there is no way you are going to get a second chance. A substantial amount of conscious effort on your part just **MAY** be able to shift the judgement. However, more often than not you would not get that opportunity as you will not be aware of what they were thinking in the first place.

So, to get the outcome you want, my advice is to do your best to ensure that the initial impression that you make is the **right** one – that is the one **you** would want.

the corporate image

To a client, or indeed anyone, who only knows *you*, *you* are the organisation.

Ensure that your image endorses how the-powers-that-be want the organisation to be seen – with a slight degree of individuality thrown in!

empathy

An empathetic image is a distinct advantage when dealing with clients or indeed with others within your own organisation.

If you look like someone's 'kind of person' you will begin at a higher level of trust/ confidence/understanding and therefore communicate more easily and more positively.

A *typical* IT boffin would not appear to be terribly empathetic to a *typical* sporty, Health Club manager; A *typical* Creative Director in an ad agency would not seem to have a natural empathy with a *typical* traditional City Banker *but who may be an important client.*

Consider carefully what this means.

Q)   If your clients are scruffy or always dressed very casually, do you really need to look like them in order to build rapport and a relationship?

A)   A most resounding "No!"

However, it would be expedient to not look *super* smart when meeting them but convey your level of empathy through what you say and do.

the importance of *your* **image** ...
... as a means to **achievement**

the look of success

Looking *successful* breeds further success.

There is no doubt that if you look successful you will be viewed as successful. I am sure that you would prefer to do business with a person, or a company, that seem to be frequently chosen and therefore approved by others.

Appearing *successful* implicitly implies that you are good at what you do.

climbing the success ladder faster

Others with the same skills and ability as yourself *but who already look the part* may well receive the next opportunity or promotion.

The advice often given is to look the part of the one immediately superior to you. If you do achieve this, there cannot be an issue about whether you look appropriate when the time comes for promotion. You obviously do.

It will also help to get you noticed at the outset.

At Positive Presence, organisations send us men or women who are being groomed for greater things but whose image is not compatible with that required at higher levels. However, in other organisations, or in other circumstances, the decision-makers may not have the inclination to invest in their employees in this way.

Get it right *yourself* now and ensure that you are first in line for the next opportunity.

increasing confidence

If every day could be a 'Look Good: Feel Good' day, think how much less stressful and better your business life would be!

I would be very surprised if you do not admit that you **feel** good when you know you **look** good. On those days, we often seem to get on swimmingly with others and everything seems easier. Accordingly, we get better results. Actually, this is because when we have more confidence, our body language and our general aura are more comfortable and in turn, this brings out the best in others.

Ultimately easier communication brings about better relationships and also leads to a more confident and enhanced performance which undoubtedly eventually increases chances of business success and promotion.

being taken seriously

Irrespective of their image, anyone who thinks, or appears, negatively is rarely viewed positively by others.

When it comes to **Presence**, (also commonly known as Impact, Credibility, Gravitas or Visibility) pale grey is an apt graphic description of someone with almost zero presence – i.e. someone who will not really be noticed or remembered. Remember, 'positive' doesn't mean just standing out; it means being noted, listened to, taken seriously and remembered for **positive** qualities, attitudes and ability.

You can measure **Presence** as a percentage. To be seen as Positive, you should aim for at least 75%.

getting the best out of life

If you make the most of yourself as far as your appearance is concerned, more often than not, you will get the best out of people and situations.

I am not talking about sexual chemistry or beauty but of portraying a well groomed, well co-ordinated, "successful" overall appearance which generates innate respect in others. This is no longer a premise but has been borne out by modern psychological research.

Even at the very beginning of life, it has been proven that pretty babies are talked to more by their mothers and by their siblings!

Besides image being important per se, the *right* business image can contribute a great deal to your career development.

the ingredients that make up
your **image**

There are several elements about *you* that together create the perception. From now on, we shall call them the Image Ingredients.

your appearance

your clothes

Your clothes are important for several reasons. When right, the feel, the cut and the look of them makes you feel good and when you are comfortable and not constrained, it shows positively in your body language.

Everything in your working wardrobe should always be comfortable, flattering – and appropriate to the situation in hand.

For peace of mind, you should aim for *your* Wardrobe to Work for *you*. When your wardrobe works, your clothes answer all your needs and you will feel comfortable and complimented by everything within it. You therefore can get on with the important things in your life in the knowledge that you know what to wear and how to wear it.

Wardrobe is very, very important but only as a complement to the other Image Ingredients.

Everybody always centres immediately on clothes when thinking about Image. A popular fantasy is that if you dress head to toe in Armani, you would look a million dollars. The sad truth is that you may not look any different than in your own High Street suit – and you will be a lot poorer! The answer is in how you choose your suit, how you apply the Finishing Touch – fit, co-ordinate, accessorise appropriately – and then ensure you complete the picture with top-to-toe grooming.

Then, if you so choose, you could still buy in the High Street – but look and feel a million dollars whilst having saved a small fortune.

your grooming

Overall, this should give an impression of cleanliness and impeccability, and shows that you care about how you look. It also says that we respect ourselves – and others – by displaying attention to detail.

Top-to-toe Grooming includes nails and hands, hair, skin (make-up *for women),* smell/ hygiene, glasses/lenses, and teeth.

your presentation

your voice

This can dispel an image or, equally, can endorse it.

This is not about accent but about voice, pitch, speed, tone, inflexion, timing and content. A high-pitched squeaky voice indicates a nervous, flibberty gibbert kind of person. Certainly not one you would want to meet on many occasions, or have confidence in in business. A slow monotone with little change in pitch would seem to belong to a slow plodding person with little personality or 'oomph' – as well as boring their audience to tears!

Voice is therefore important in contributing to the actual image of the owner. However, a pleasant and interesting voice is always a plus factor. People enjoy listening to it and the added benefit is that they pay greater attention – and accordingly remember more about what you say.

your non-verbal behaviour

Face and body language tells us a great deal about a person but often without us realising it at a conscious level. When we begin to look better – and therefore feel better – about ourselves, these messages often change positively as they are basically reflectors of our own confidence and self-image.

your manners, etiquette and behaviour

The need for manners and etiquette is sometimes said to be fast disappearing in the modern world. Personally, I believe that it is best to conform as it is still considered by many as most important. If you are not seen to practise this code, it could certainly count against you in certain situations. So, it is always best to know what is viewed as right and then at least you can make an *informed* decision about whether to use it or not.

Manners and etiquette are also a means of showing respect to others and that can certainly do no harm as long as it is not seen to be overdone, sycophantic or old fashioned.

Behaviour is somewhat different and should always be congruent with the image you are choosing to portray. For example, to project an image of maturity, authority and responsibility, an up-and-coming executive would be better not seen chewing gum, drinking Coke and reading comics!

summary

The Importance of Image

AS A COMMUNICATION TOOL

It sends out messages about you.

If the FIRST IMPRESSION isn't *right*, you rarely get the chance to make a second.

Empathy expedites business relationships.

You are the corporate image – that is a position of responsibility in itself.

AS A MEANS TO ACHIEVEMENT

A POSITIVE PRESENCE will be treated positively.

Appearing "successful" means, in crude terms that people *buy* you. You   must be good at what you do. Others will therefore want you too!

Attractive people generally get the best out of people and situations.

Looking the part of your superior may well aid climbing the ladder faster.

The Image Ingredients

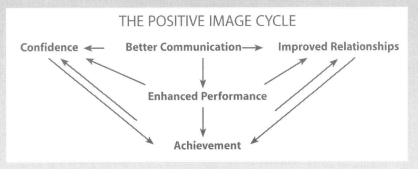

THE POSITIVE IMAGE CYCLE

Confidence ←— Better Communication —→ Improved Relationships

Enhanced Performance

Achievement

APPEARANCE

Wardrobe and Good Grooming

PRESENTATION

Voice and Content, Body Language, Manners, Etiquette and Behaviour

notes

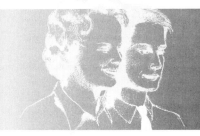

laying the foundations

So far, we have explored why this subject is so important to you and your career and how messages about you are transmitted by your overall image and by each Image Ingredient.

Now we must decide on our objective and assess what and how much needs to be addressed.

Thinking about your **present** image

Watch TV and particularly observe the commercials. TV time costs serious money and so the images you see instantly create an impression in order that you identify with the subject – and buy the product!

Think about typical images which relate to:

- A suburban middle-class (wo)man

- A City Investment Banker

- A tea lady

- A successful, sophisticated European business(wo)man

- A University student

- An Oxford/Cambridge professor

How might they look and sound?

Similarly, we instantly recognise stereotypes in real life and respond accordingly. If we relate to it, we 'buy' the product.

Think of *you* or *your service* as the product!

How do you look and sound? Would people recognise you for what you are?

Thinking about your **aspired** image

You need to think hard about what the right image is for you, the necessity to achieve it and to commit to it. You should not even think of changing radically overnight. For this to really work, it must be a gradual development, a type of metamorphosis. It needs to be an evolution, not a revolution. As changes take place, you will feel good about yourself, especially if you are complimented by others. As you get used to the change and feel comfortable with it, you will feel ready to take even more on board in a way that you were not at first.

To help you consider Business Image in a new light, fill in answers to the questions on Table-2.

table 2	
your business image	
in which way would a successful *(whatever you do)* be portrayed in a TV play/film/ad?	
how you recognise business and professional people as successful?	
if appropriate, give adjectives that describe your company or organisation's corporate image?	
which of the above apply to you?	
which do not – but should?	
look at your superiors again. Do they look better than you – if so, in which ways?	
what percentage of your working days are 'Look Good:Feel Good' days?	

testing opinion

1. *your* presence

Think of people you know in shades of grey.

Those with a really strong Presence will be so grey that they will be black.

Those with a low rating will probably be hard to recall.

Ask three people who know you to assess your Presence on a zero to 100% rating – or in terms of grey – and complete Table 3.

table 3										
greyish white		**pale grey**		**mid-grey**		**dark grey**		**almost black**		
0	**10**	**20**	**30**	**40**	**50**	**60**	**70**	**80**	**90**	**100%**
your **presence**		**SCORE 1**	**%**			**SCORE 2**	**%**		**SCORE 3**	**%**

Add together your scores and divide by three to calculate your current Presence factor.

testing opinion

2. *your* PRESENT IMAGE

Image is not the way that you believe you portray yourself to others.

It is others' perception of you.

To give you a framework within which to work, we need to test both how you see yourself and how you are seen by others.

Use Table 4 below to record the answers for future reference.

- Enter five adjectives (keywords) that currently describe your Present business image.

- Enter five adjectives (keywords) that *you would like* to describe your business image. i.e. your Aspired business image.

- Now you need to test others opinions. If possible, it would be sensible to incorporate someone else's help to organise this and then compile the list without you knowing who said what. This would remove any bias in the answers from people who do not wish to offend you.

- Ask the following groups to choose five adjectives that describe your business image and add them to the table.
  Three business colleagues/contacts who do not know you very well.
  Three business colleagues/contacts who do know you well.
  Three of your work superiors.
  Three others who only know you by telephone.

Compare the adjectives in each set with each other and then with the other groups. You can now draw your own conclusions about how you are perceived by others.

table 4				
keywords		1	2	3
your **present** image				
colleagues who don't know you very well	1			
	2			
	3			
those who know you only by phone	1			
	2			
	3			
colleagues who know you well	1			
	2			
	3			
superiors	1			
	2			
	3			
your **aspired** image				

4	5	your conclusions

testing opinion

3. *your* image ingredients

Ask your family, colleagues and friends about your voice, your smile, eye contact, facial expressions, general demeanour, posture, walk, handshake and your appearance i.e. grooming and clothes.

Record the answers on Table 5 so that you can refer to them from time to time as we work through the Image Ingredients.

table 5		
what they say		
voice		
facial expression		
demeanour		
posture		
walk		
handshake		
smile		
eye contact		
grooming and clothes		

WARNING! This should only be used as a guide as some comments may be totally subjective.

...continued		
voice		
facial expression		
demeanour		
posture		
walk		
handshake		
smile		
eye contact		
grooming and clothes		

self assessment

1. Using the questions below as a prompt, take a realistic and relevant standard and assess yourself on Table 6 with regard to each Image Ingredient.

2. Identify the reasons why you think you haven't worked on remedying this before – i.e. consider your own 'obstacles'.

1. wardrobe

Does *your* Wardrobe Work for *you*?

It should contain. . .

- Something appropriate for every normal occasion in your life such as conferences, meetings, weddings, funerals, dinners, etc. so that you don't need to rush out and panic buy.

- Many combinations so that you never feel bored.

- Versatile garments that can be adapted from day to evening and work to leisure.

- A capsule travelling wardrobe so that packing is a pleasure, not a chore.

- Flattering, comfortable clothes that make you feel and look good.

- Only clothes that you actually wear.

2. voice and verbal contents

What does your voice imply about you . . . is it pleasant to listen to?

Tape yourself and listen carefully. Can you be clearly understood?

Consider whether people seem generally to understand easily what you are trying to tell them.

- Do they listen and take notice?

- Do you get the result you want?

- Do they get impatient?

- Do they remember what you say?

- Do you manage to persuade and to influence easily?

3. non-verbal

What messages can you spot about yourself that you may previously not have been aware of?

Get out a few photographs and a recent video and critically observe yourself.

Sit, stand and move in front of a mirror and think about how you look, how you sit, how you gesticulate etc.

4. grooming

Take a long hard and honest look at yourself.

Overall, do you appear . . .

Immaculate?	Modern?
Well Groomed?	Fit and healthy?

You have now given some thought to how you believe you are perceived by others.

You have also tested to what extent you were correct. Having worked out what you would like your image to be, you can use the information that you have collected.

This should help greatly towards understanding what exactly you need to do to meet your goal.

table 6	
image – self assessment	
image ingedient	**1 your assessment of your current standard**
voice	1
	2
facial expression	1
	2
demeanour	1
	2
posture	1
	2
walk	1
	2
handshake	1
	2
smile	1
	2
eye contact	1
	2
appearance	1
	2
grooming	1
	2
wardrobe	1
	2

2 your reasons for not having worked on this before

summary

Think about your Image:

> **Present**
>
> **Aspired**

Test Opinion regarding your:

> **Business Image**
>
> **Image Ingredients**
>
> **Presence**

Self-Assessment (honest!)

What were the obstacles that stopped you making changes before now?
(Again, you may need to do some soul searching!)

notes

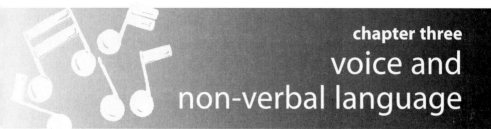

We shall now begin all the necessary work on your Image Ingredients. Knowing that your presentation is an integral part of your image, we shall discover what you can do to improve it.

I was recently invited to talk to a very important group of engineers who I assumed would be cynical about the importance of image. I therefore had to decide on a strategy that would make the necessary initial impact. Instead of arriving and pre-networking with the guests, I was hidden in an anteroom and, when announced, I *scurried* in. After being introduced by way of a high-profile build up, I began to talk in a high pitched, squeaky and breathless voice, allowing my words to trip over themselves. Meanwhile, I maintained a hunched shoulder posture and gesticulated wildly. After two or three sentences, I sat down abruptly to a horrified silence.

At this point, my observers would have assumed me to be scatty, nervous, unconfident, untidy, etc. Certainly not a successful entrepreneur or recognised image guru! Although this judgement would have come primarily from my voice, my posture and body language would have further endorsed it.

Conversely, had I have sloped in and droned in a flat monotone whilst staring fixedly at my audience, they would have switched off pretty quickly. In this instance, they would have assessed me as someone slow, boring, uninspiring, personality-less, dull and ordinary; again, most certainly not dynamic, inspirational, motivational or of leadership calibre.

After a few seconds, I rose again and, standing quite upright with hands neatly by my side, clearly engaging my audience with good eye contact and a genuine smile, I addressed them in my normal, *hopefully* pleasant and well-modulated, voice:

".................... Gentlemen, *that* is the power of **Image!**"

the voice

Academic research proves that 38% of the impression you make comes from the way that you sound whilst only 7% from what you actually say.

Be aware of the power of your voice and how you can use it to advantage.

In business terms, your voice should convey that you are:

* Informed
* Confident
* Responsible
* Authoritative
* In control
* Sensible
* Reliable
* Sincere
* Energised
* Competent

YOUR VOICE	
should be	**should** *not* **be**
pleasant	rasping
interesting	squeaky
energised	booming
communicative	dull
convincing	monotonous
	mumbling

the voice variables

Sincerity	Sound like *you* believe in what you say – or *they* won't
Clarity	Enunciate so that your words are heard clearly
Breathing	Listeners should not be aware of your breath – or lack of it
Pause	Use frequently to aid absorption and comprehension
Passion	Sound like *you* care – or *they* won't
Inflexion	Use emphasis and "throwaway" remarks
Pace	Don't leave them behind ... or let them race ahead of you
Pitch	Move up and down the octave for maximum impact
Tone	Select the appropriate one – critical, angry, sympathetic, etc.
Humour	Lightens the load but can subtly emphasise the message
Volume	Be sure you can be heard – but not *over*heard

Accents add variation and can induce interest. However, do listeners often ask you to repeat yourself? If so, it means you are not easily understood by your clarity, your pace . . . or your accent.

Think also about "sounds" like grunts, clearing your throat, a nervous cough, 'ums' and 'ahs', a lisp, grinding teeth, etc *and what they convey.*

non-verbal behaviour

NON-VERBAL BEHAVIOUR is how we send messages in all the other ways besides what we say. It tells us a great deal about a person – but almost always subconsciously – **which means that we make judgements – and often without realising it.**

To ensure that you are being read as you would like, you need to check yourself out. The best way is to conduct research amongst friends and colleagues. Also ask people at work who hardly know you.

Actually, they are the most valuable of all.

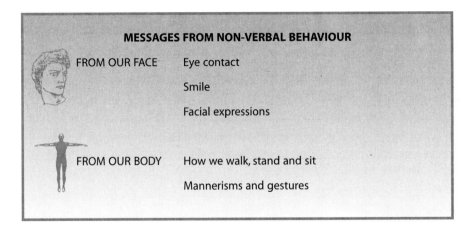

MESSAGES FROM NON-VERBAL BEHAVIOUR

FROM OUR FACE   Eye contact

                         Smile

                         Facial expressions

FROM OUR BODY   How we walk, stand and sit

                         Mannerisms and gestures

the way we look

Our face is probably the most telling as it is usually the point of focus.

The expression "eyes are the mirror of our soul," says everything. *Normal* eye contact, as opposed to a false fixed level, puts people at their ease – as does a warm, genuine and frequent (but not too frequent!) smile.

Our overall facial expression should be relaxed. Tensing of various muscles demonstrates tension, anxiety, stress etc. e.g. winces, frowns, pursing lips, screwing up eyes, biting lips, clenching jaw.

	action	message you are sending about yourself
blinking rate	Accelerated blinking pattern	*Nervous disposition*
eye contact	Fixed penetrating stare into recipients eyes	*I'm not letting you get away*
		I am supercilious / controlling
	Avoiding eyes by looking everywhere else	*I can't be trusted*
smile	The "Salesman" – a fixed smile that does not come from the eyes	*I don't mean a word of it*
	A short smile delivered at the end of almost every sentence	*I am very unsure of myself*
facial expressions	Clenching jaw	*I am worried*
	Puckered or pursed lips	*I don't understand*
	Twitches	*I am not confident*
	Frown	*I am stressed*
	Screwed up eyes	*I am of nervous disposition*
	Tense lips set in tight line	*I am scared*
	Frequent blinking	*I can't cope*
	Licking/Biting/ Chewing lips	

Mr. A(Anxious) came in to discuss how best he could provide his service to a major corporate. Throughout the meeting, although feeling quite confident, he wore a worried look, frowning often, as this was his natural disposition.

Mr. S(Salesman) came next, smiling a great deal but with a clenched jaw and eyes that were narrowed and cold.

He was followed by Mr. C (Confident), another competitor, who appeared to be well at ease, smiling genuinely when necessary and ensuring normal eye contact with the interviewer.

Who would you choose?

Mary noticed that people were always saying to her "Cheer up love; it may never happen!" or asking her "What's the matter?"
She finally twigged that she had a naturally unhappy expression.
She learned to look happier, less tense and smile more.
Result: Mary actually feels happier and more positive.
She also gets better results in all aspects of her life.

In any selection process like a job interview or tendering for business, displaying anxiety or lack of confidence can never be in your favour. It will obviously make others think that *you yourself* don't believe that *you* can deliver what is required. If *you* don't, how can *they*?

the way we move

The authoritative person will make smoother, open, more regular movements whilst the less confident one will make jerky ones and hold their arms more tightly into the body.

standing

We use Posture like a mask. It also can easily become a habit sending out the wrong messages about how you are really feeling at the time.

How much straighter and better we stand when we are dressed up or how we steel ourselves for something unpleasant by squaring our shoulders? We use our posture everyday without realising it and, by the same token, we read the signals in other people without them having to utter a word.

When you are feeling tired, you slouch and droop. This also tends to happen when you don't feel confident and, if this is usual for you, the slouch can easily become your natural stance.

Similarly, when you are angry you will lean slightly forward with your shoulders rising up towards your ears. If you tend often to feel angry or "put out", this will certainly reflect in your posture – and may become a habit.

Your positioning in relation to others needs also to be considered. Crowding in on someone's space can make them feel intimidated and overwhelmed. On the other hand, standing too far apart can be seen to convey aloofness. When you feel unsure, gauge what is best by watching carefully how others are reacting to the space between you.

good posture

- Stand with feet side by side
- Keep legs straight but not tense
- Breathe slowly and evenly
- Roll your shoulders back
- Lift chin slightly
- Imagine that puppet strings are holding up your head
- Your weight should be just forward of centre

walking

Your walk illustrates how you command space and this usually reflects the extent to which one commands in other aspects of life too.

An assertive, purposeful person will take longer, slower and more definite strides. A meeker, less confident counterpart may scurry or, conversely, plod or shuffle.

sitting

You should sit squarely and neatly, not slouch or sprawl, with your back firmly parallel to the back of the chair and with your legs folded or crossed tidily

Your arms should be folded loosely on your lap – *not* folded tightly against your chest which may say: *"I won't let you in; I'm not open to ideas"; or "Don't mess with me".*

> **I was invited to sit in on an assessment panel for appointing a CEO to a local government position. I certainly won't forget the candidate who slouched to one side of his chair, leaning on his elbow which was splayed out on the arm of the chair throughout the interview. His whole manner displayed arrogance, even contempt, which was finally endorsed when he patronisingly complimented the interviewer on her quality of question!**

mannerisms, gestures and actions

Subtle messages can be sent through all mannerisms, gestures and actions but your handshake is a major contributor to 'their' First Impression of you.

		no	yes
handshake		**The Wet Fish** A floppy soft hand gingerly offered	**A firm grasp with 3 or 4 regular up-and-down movements**
		The Pump A resounding attempt to break your arm	

Possible implications – dishonesty etc.

- Fiddling with nails, objects etc.

- Flicking or touching hair

- Constantly touching, rubbing, pulling any facial feature

- Crossing and uncrossing legs

- Shifting from side to side

- Hand shielding front of face

- Rubbing hands together

Possible implications – impatience etc.

- Crossing and uncrossing legs

- Foot and finger tapping

- Folding and unfolding arms

- Head resting on hand

- Shrugs

Remember too, repeated mannerisms and gestures can prove intensely irritating to others.

Before we consider your appearance, you need to work on your voice and your facial and body language. Seriously take into account what you discovered from testing others' opinions and from your own observations. If you feel that you really need more help, there are professionals who coach in these specialist areas, including Positive Presence, of course.

summary

Your presentation consists of three different elements
- **your Voice**
- **your Non-Verbal Language**
- **your Manners, Etiquette and Behaviour**

Each one is important on their own merit but *collectively* they send out even more powerful messages about you

notes

_____

_____

_____

_____

_____

_____

_____

_____

_____

_____

_____

_____

good grooming

One of our main problems in the UK is the lack of emphasis on good grooming. It is generally believed – and propounded further by the media – that business image is fundamentally about the clothes that you wear.

However if the grooming and the finishing touches are dealt with so that they send a positive message, you can get away with a great deal less in the wardrobe department.

It is my belief that there is something in the British culture that has made it difficult for us to accept that appearance should be a priority. On the Continent, it is usually considered the normal way of life. Just like they enjoy *good* food and wine everyday – not just on high days and holidays. It has been proven beyond doubt that people enjoy, and respond positively to, attractive people in the same way as they do to art, architecture, music and surroundings that are pleasing to the eye and ear. It must therefore be in order to make ourselves as attractive as possible, both for ourselves and to obtain the most positive reaction we can from others.

good grooming

Hair	**Skin (incl. Make-up)**
Nails and hands	**Smell**
Eyewear	**Teeth**
Jewellery	**Accessories**

hair on the head

Your hair is one of the most important Image Ingredients and it should be your crowning glory.

Hair should always be clean, tidy, healthy and glossy. Over-greasy hair should be washed daily but use a gentle shampoo (for 'frequent use') and forget the old wives tale that it will fall out! For flyaway hair, use conditioner afterwards and wash out well or use a leave-in one that is specially formulated.

As far as hair for business is concerned, there are three basic requirements:

- Your hair needs to look good *everyday*, not just when you have extra time or make a special effort.

- The style should endorse your credibility in your business role.

- Your hair shape and colouring should be flattering to your face, your body and your proportions.

common excuses for a 'bad hair day'

"It was the rain, the sun, the wind etc.

The heat always does this

I didn't have enough time this morning

I'm overdue for a visit to the hairdresser

My hair always needs 2 or 3 days to settle after it's cut

I'm growing my hair out

It was a mistake by the hairdresser"

There should *never* be any need for excuses to others ... or to yourself.

The best advice for you is to **try a new hairdresser now** (even though that may not be what you want to hear!)

I know that you may like the familiarity of someone you are used to but it is quite likely to be a false economy. Try going up a notch or two; get it cut really well and then see and feel if there is a difference. A good cut is essential in creating a shape that looks good *everyday* with very little attention.

Ask around to find a recommended hairdresser who, besides being skilled at their trade, will understand your lifestyle and its demands. A new hairdresser will be able to look at you objectively as you are only an image to him/her at that point, rather than a person. Ask them to describe what they would suggest *if* they were given carte blanche. Also ask his/her advice on how to maintain your new style and the best products to use.

Then, if you feel unsure or resistant, I would advise you to compromise but take into account the following criteria:

- **Your normal regime**
  Whether you are office based, mobile, travel, entertain clients etc.

- **Time *and your level of inclination* to look after your hair**

- **Appropriateness to your job**

Women: Long hair is always going to look more business-like if neatly worn back and up (but not in a ponytail!).

Men: Similarly, in traditional sectors, length should not hang over the collar. NB Re spiky and untidy fashionable styles: I am often asked whether these are deemed appropriate for business. Whilst this is fashionable, I would suggest it best to be expedient in the more traditional sectors like finance, health and law, and take geographical factors into account too. You would be best advised to carefully consider your role, the sector and the working environment. If still in doubt, take the less risky option. However, if this is of great importance to you, ask your hairdresser for a style that answers all the necessary criteria but that can also be adjusted to the look you like in your private life. And then ensure that you know how to **do** it yourself.

- **Your age**

Women: I am often asked about the suitability of long hair over 40. I believe that most women approaching mid-life are more flattered by shorter hair diverting the eye up away from the areas that are naturally going down!

Men: Just be careful that you don't look like an ageing hippie!

- **The proportion of the size of your head to your body**
  If you can, you should add or remove width or height to balance with the rest of the body. However, sometimes there are other factors! In the case of men or women who are very thin on top, there's really *nothing* that you can do with the size of your head, only with your body!

- **Your face and features**
  The face shape, angularity and fullness, the ears, nose, eyes, forehead etc.

- **Hair type:**
  Texture – coarse, fine or normal
  Inclination – curly, wavy straight
  Abundance – thick, thin or normal

Especially for Men: A note on receding hair Unfortunately there is still no miracle cure although many are advertised and marketed voraciously. My best advice is to accept what is happening in good spirit and concentrate on maximising all your other attributes. Please do not be drawn into brushing a few lonely strands forward to try to disguise the thinning patch or to even think about wearing a toupée. Console yourself in the knowledge that it is cool to be bald and many women find it extremely sexy!

Especially for Women: A note on colour I would suggest that once you have dealt with your make-up, you take a new look at your hair colour in relation to your current skin tone. Your hair should provide a definite and flattering contrast to your complexion.

In the case of the not quite so young, hair usually fades as time marches on, as does skin. It can subtly add interest to have lowlights or highlights. Strategically placed, they emphasise good features or divert from the negative ones whilst also making the hair look thicker by adding texture and by giving a three dimensional effect.

hair on the face

Men   Undoubtedly, as facial hair is a controversial issue, it would seem prudent to just conform and be clean-shaven. Even so, it must be said that Designer stubble and other facial hair may be highly acceptable – even desirable! – in creative, IT and other such sectors. You have to weigh up the balance between what, where and when it is acceptable – and just looking plain unkempt!

However, another aspect to take into account is that moustaches and beards are considered predominant features and are therefore those by which you would be described or remembered.

If you have good features, why not let others notice those instead? I have had so many instances where removing facial hair provokes appreciative comments – certainly ones about looking younger.

If you are blessed with bushy eyebrows, they will grow bushier and closer together in time – remember Denis Healey? They can be easily pruned with the razor or waxed by your local beautician.

One last word. Without question hair that is visible in the ears or nostrils is unsightly – and ageing.

Women   Please check that none is visible. A visit to your local beautician can deal with it very effectively and should be considered of the highest priority.

teeth

Smile as often as genuinely possible to reveal *perfect* teeth. If they are not even or white, visit the dentist and consider some cosmetic dentistry such as straightening, whitening, veneers or professional cleaning by the hygienist.

eyewear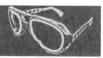

Unfortunately for all who wear them, glasses are now a fashion item that are costly and date very quickly.

you need to make sure that ...

- *You* wear *them – they* don't wear *you*

- **They suit your face, body and image**
  Experiment with all types of different styles using a friend or   colleague as a sounding board.

- **You buy something that won't date too quickly**
  By observing others, watching TV and looking at magazines you should get an idea of what is really old-fashioned but also what may be 'here today, gone tomorrow'.

- **They fit you**
  They should not be wider than your face or hide your eyebrow. They should not rest on your cheeks, as constantly pushing them on your nose, often unconsciously, can be irritating and distractive to others.

If you wear lenses, check that you wear them unobtrusively. Bulging eyes – or ever-blinking ones – are not attractive.

glasses – the choices

Frames	Lenses
Round or angular lines	Rims or rimless
Thick or thin rims	Tinted or opaque lenses
Large or small	Shaded or uniform lenses
Metal or other materials	Plastic or glass lenses
The colouring	Special light-changing feature

nails and hands

Hands should always look clean and well cared for. Hand creams are readily available that moisturise the hands and nourish the nails.

Nails should be clean, smooth and well shaped. Bitten nails are *never* acceptable – besides looking unsightly, they demonstrate nervousness and inability to cope under pressure.

Cuticles should be neat and soft. If they appear scraggy or over thick, push them down with an orange stick and apply a little cuticle cream nightly.

Manicures – for both sexes – are often considered a really enjoyable and inexpensive treat.

<table>
<tr><td>

BEWARE

The HR Manager of a leading City Investment bank told me that bitten nails are one of the first things they spot – and then they automatically reject the owner.

</td><td>

TIP

A mixture of sugar and washing-up liquid rubbed in well and then washed away will remove any ingrained grease, paint, dye or oil.

</td></tr>
</table>

Women: Nails should have some length, be filed into an attractive rounded shape, but not look like talons.

Always use polish to some degree. Whether a soft pale pink, a French manicure or a more pronounced yet muted tone, a varnished nail demonstrates attention to detail, feminising and a personal touch to the work "uniform". Shocking pink, bright red etc. could be deemed inappropriate, as would finishes such as blue, mauve, sparkles etc.

For a professional finish, always use a base coat and a topcoat.

smell

We should always smell fresh and clean. As I often have to deal with these ever so sensitive problems in my day-to-day work, I would like to briefly bring them to your attention for you to consider whether any could apply to you.

underarm

A deodorant is essential together with an eau de cologne/after-shave for men and perfume/eau de toilette for women. There is unlimited choice of scents, growing by the week, and so much depends on your own personal preference. Choose something that is personally pleasing, pleasant and present to others whilst not overpowering.

CASE STUDY

Recently I was asked to deal with a senior Bank Manager who didn't smell as he should – particularly on a hot summer's day. It was so bad that his secretary had left and the current one was thinking of following the same course. Hints had been made but fallen on deaf ears. Had it remained unchecked, it would have had a detrimental effect on the man's career and limit his promotional prospects.

However a few direct words in his ear resulted in a happy ending.

hair and skin

should *smell* fresh and clean as well as appear so.

feet

can smell very cheesy. You can easily test by sniffing your shoes and socks/stockings when you take them off. It is easy to buy shoe, feet and hosiery deodorants and ensure that you air your shoes – and never wear them two days running.

underwear and clothes

absorb body, cooking and smoking odours and must be washed or dry-cleaned regularly.

breath

is another area of which to be most conscious.

These are things that most of us take for granted. However, if everyone knew and practiced them, there just wouldn't be any need to comment on them!

skincare for men

Today the mens' cosmetic market is worth billions of pounds and growing day by day as men realise the importance of looking after their skin. Many ranges are available now which are especially formulated for men such as Clinique, Boots and Clarins.

Skin should always look healthy, unblemished, clean and with an even colour.

Dead cells can make the skin surface uneven so exfoliating once or twice a week keeps it looking alive. Greasy skin can be helped by the regular use of facemasks and tonic to cleanse and close pores.

Good shaving is essential to the appearance of your skin.

before shaving

Wait at least half an hour after you get up in the morning to allow facial muscles to tighten and give whiskers a chance to stand away from the skin.

Wash first with warm water to remove dirt and grime and soften bristles. This also improves razor glide as the texture of beard hair is like that of copper wire.

Massage in your chosen shaving cream to lubricate the skin and soften the beard.

shaving

Always soften with warm water before shaving – it's often a good idea to shave in the shower.

Shave jawline and cheeks first, then neck, upper and lower lips and lastly the chin, where the whiskers are the thickest.

Shave in the direction of the natural beard growth – don't go against the grain!

Rinse your razor often to prevent clogging. As shaving can remove three skin layers, don't shave over the same spot several times.

Wet shaving is kinder to the skin, though on a regular basis it may be irritating to men with dry or sensitive skin who should consider alternating electric and wet shaving.

Prepare the bristles for a more comfortable electric shave with a Pre-Electric Shave product which improves the movement of the shaver to help prevent razor burn.

and after ...

Splash your face with warm water. Gently pat dry with a soft, clean towel.

Soothe and lightly moisturise skin. Should you feel a moisturiser leaves your skin too oily, apply an oil free gel which doesn't leave a greasy after-feel and is mildly medicated.

skincare for women

essentials

- Scrupulous cleansing.
- Exfoliate, including lips, once or twice weekly to keep skin looking alive.
- Nourish nightly to replace what is lost through ageing and the environment.
- Moisturisers should be chosen carefully on the basis of being easily absorbed and never feeling greasy.

make-up

This is one of those very controversial issues that come up time and time again. I am a believer that a woman in business should wear make–up *that is visible* as part of her groomed finished look. But 'Visible' does not mean thick, mask like or plastered on. It means flattering and used to even and enhance skin tone and facial features. And for the younger reader, although natural is 'in', there is natural – and there is natural! Much prejudice or fixed thinking actually comes from lack of real and relevant information. Just look carefully at the pretty young models and other celebs in the media. Most do wear natural, yet *visible* make-up – and look really good too!

valid – the reasons to wear visible make-up

A survey carried out recently in the USA proved that women who wear make-up earn 25% more than their counterparts who don't.

Natural is fine but invisible is not appropriate for the professional woman who needs to show that she is well groomed.

With the level of pollution and the danger from harmful UVA and UVB rays today, make-up should be considered a protection, not to the contrary.

Very few women are at their most attractive in their natural state, particularly as the years creep on. It can only make sense to use and appreciate the help that is available over the counter.

My best advice is to forget the obstacles, re-visit the whole concept with new thinking – and then commit to using Make-Up as one of your priorities. I assure you from my years of experience that the compliments that you will receive and your increased confidence will make it all worthwhile.

However, you need to achieve a make-up regime that is:

- quick
- easy
- up-to-date
- appropriate to your life
- makes you feel your best

> . . . and then practise it religiously every day until it becomes an automatic part of your daily routine

invalid – the reasons *not* to wear visible make-up

I feel uncomfortable with make-up.

Laurel's reply: If you are unused to something, you undoubtedly feel both different, and strange, when you first do it. If you had never worn glasses and then were told to, you would feel very peculiar the first week, a little less the week after and, then within a month, you would feel like you have always been wearing them. It is the same with make-up.

Everyone will notice and comment that I suddenly look different.

Laurel's reply: Anything that is different is often treated with suspicion, sometimes fear, and commented on negatively. To combat this, I would start first with a little mascara and follow with a new eyebrow shape: then a more defined lipstick shade a week later. After a little time passes, add visible foundation with some subtle blusher. Gradually you will achieve the objective without hearing comments that may undermine your confidence (but that are truly very little to do with you!).

It's too expensive

Laurel's reply: The High Street ranges are very good and reasonably priced. As you grow more confident, you can begin to experiment and invest a little more.

It takes too long in the morning

Laurel's reply: My daily make-up takes me under three minutes and certainly should take no more than five. Everyone can spare that! It's just a matter of making this a priority like brushing one's teeth or bathing.

It's too difficult and will take too much effort

Laurel's reply: Well, it won't be once you know how and what to do. Don't you feel the same with anything that is new – each new computer programme, a new car etc?

I don't know how

Laurel's reply: Well, you will by the end of this chapter!

your basic daily make-up

skin

colour correctors

If your skin tone is very uneven, very pale, sallow, blotchy, or with very high colour it will benefit from a colour corrector applied very sparingly in the relevant areas.

foundation

This should even out texture and colour but not mask or hide your skin. Most of us are best with water-based foundations that offer medium coverage.

Your foundation should be your main investment so buy carefully.

Apply small dots of foundation over your face with a cosmetic wedge, a Ramer baby sponge or a foundation brush.

Blend all over the face with downward and outward strokes and ensure it is taken out to the hairline, under the chin and fade into the neck colour. If you have used corrector, blend in at the edges but don't cover with the foundation.

Look straight ahead into a mirror facing daylight (or lit from the top at night). If you can see shadows and blemishes, you need to add a foundation in a lighter shade and gently apply it with your little finger – or a brush – on all those areas.

concealer

Where there are spots, age spots, scars or lines that still show, work in concealer very sparingly from a dab on your hand with a special concealer brush.

powder

Dip a felt powder puff in translucent loose powder and then *firmly* press into your skin, including eyelids and mouth. If you prefer a more natural look or if you have very dry skin, just powder nose, chin and forehead to reduce the shine.

Brush off excess with large clean brush or cotton wool dipped in cold water and squeezed well.

Pressed powder should only be used for topping up during the day.

blusher

Choose a tawny shade to define cheekbones and a second blush colour (amber, coral pink or dusky) to give you some natural looking colour.

Shading: Suck in cheekbones and apply shading slightly in triangle under cheekbones. Blend in very well with clean brush or powder puff.

Blush Colour: With an upward and outward motion move the brush up the apple of the cheeks to the temple to give a healthy glow and repeat until the necessary depth of colour is reached.

eyes

eyebrows

If your eyebrows are not a neat shape, pluck them or have them shaped first professionally as a guide. A good eyebrow shape frames your eye and opens it up, making it look larger and more awake.

Brush eyebrows to remove excess powder and then lightly pencil in a flattering frame for your eye. The end nearest the nose should not look too heavy and the colour chosen should be close to your natural eyebrow unless you are very fair.

eyeshadow

Load your eyeshadow brush with a lightish natural powder eyeshadow (natural looking beiges or soft greys are safest) and cover eyelid area.

Load a sponge applicator or an eyeshadow shading brush with a darker shade (Brown, grey or navy). Find the socket line; sweep this on and above this line to create an arc. Blend well with a clean brush.

eyeliner

Use a pencil or eyeshadow on a very fine brush to line your upper and lower eyelids – dry for softness, wet for stronger definition. Dot initially and then smudge together.

Only take line three quarters of the way towards inner corners if your eyes are set close together.

mascara

Optional: Use eyelash curlers *first.*

Apply one or two coats of mascara allowing each to dry thoroughly before applying the next, and then use a special lash comb to separate the lashes.

lips

Using a tissue, blot lips to remove any excess grease.

With a sharpened lip pencil, or lip brush loaded with slightly darker colour lipstick, draw a neat line around the edge of lips using short strokes. You can adjust your own lipline slightly if necessary.

Powder to set the line and fill in with your chosen shade, blending it with the line.

Using your tissue, blot and apply a second coat.

Always touch up your make-up in the middle of the day

... and refresh in the evening.

make-up tips

* Buy very good brushes that you can control.

* Clean your brushes in soapy water once a week and let them dry naturally.

* Don't hoard foundation; when it separates it has turned rancid. Bin it.

* Use a lipbrush to use up lipstick to the very bottom.

* Use a cleaned mascara wand from a finished mascara to brush eyebrows and separate lashes.

* If you were ever talked into buying transparent mascara (a real con!), it can be used up as a finishing gel for eyebrows.

* The best time to apply moisturiser to your face is before a bath as the steam helps it to penetrate your skin.

* When buying foundation:
    Go with naked skin.
    Select 2 or 3 shades nearest to your jaw and neck colour.
    Always check in daylight.
    Also buy another, one shade lighter, for shading together with a concealer to match.

* You can apply dark brown or grey eyeshadow with a fine brush for a very natural looking eyebrow.

* Blend a tiny dot of concealer on the outside corner of your eye where the top and bottom lashes meet and see how wide-awake you look.

* In hot weather, store cosmetic pencils in fridge before sharpening to prevent them breaking.

- For a more natural look, wipe the mascara wand with a tissue to remove excess.

- For lip colour that fades, try a fixative or fill in lips entirely with pencil before applying lipstick. Blot and powder lightly. Repeat two or three times.

- For compressed powders, e.g. blusher or eyeshadow, load brush first, i.e. sweep the brush over palette and then tap several times to remove excess colour.

survival kit

- Clinique Turnaround 15 minute facial.

- Touche Éclat (Radiant Touch) by YSL – marvellous for tired shadows under eyes and fine lines.

- Flash Balm by Clarins wakes up tired looking skin.

- Issima Midnight Secret by Guerlain makes you look like you have had a good night's sleep – even with a heavy hangover.

- Dr Nelson eye mask.

- Elizabeth Arden 8-Hour Cream – great for dry skin. Can also be used as a conditioner for lips.

- Jurlique Herbal Recovery Gel – a non-surgical lift that is totally organic.

- Use a little moisturiser to thin out too heavy foundation or to deal with cakey concealer.

- Use loose powder to reduce too much blusher, too-dark eyeshadow or too-hard looking eyeliner.

- Use a cotton bud with a small amount of non-oily eye make-up remover to remove smudges. Re-apply foundation and powder to re-set.

- Clean up a smudged lip line with a cotton bud dipped in make-up remover. Re-apply foundation then re-define lip border and powder.

We have now addressed all the aspects of grooming to give you an immaculate, fit and energised business image.

Grooming is very important but you must get the clothes 100% right as well.

summary

Top-to-toe grooming is key

    Hair

    Smell

    Teeth

    Skincare

    Nails and hands

    Shaving for men

    Eyewear if relevant

    Make-up for women

notes

chapter five
the business wardrobe

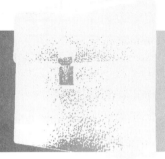

A positive business image conveys you are:

Competent	Professional
On the leading edge	Open, friendly, approachable
Organised	Attention to detail
Successful	Sensible
Relevant	Committed to your work

We have now sorted out your grooming, and emphasised its importance.

Your hair, skin, nails, hands and teeth all *look* absolutely spot-on! Your skin, hair, body and breath should *smell* just as good!

Now we can get on to your upholstery – that is, your clothes! However, this is a really, really, big subject and there are many variables which serve to confuse rather than to clarify. We must begin by considering what Business Wear consists of in general terms which will help you to identify what it means for you.

A *positive* business image is conveyed when your clothes are always:

- **Immaculate**
- **Contemporary**
- **Stylish**
- **Appropriate**

- **Immaculate**

    Well-pressed, tidy, spotless, hemlines even, no threads hanging and buttons
    secured, no dandruff or stray hairs on collar or shoulders.

- **Contemporary**

Not old fashioned – but certainly doesn't have to mean up-to-the-minute.

- **Stylish**

To be Stylish is to be aware of fashion but not be controlled by it.

> *Fashion is what we're given; Style is what we choose*
> *Fashion is today; Style is yesterday, today and tomorrow*
> *Style is about confidence; not about cash*

- **Appropriate to . . .**

    the sector
    There are some like the City, the education, creative and voluntary
    sectors that most definitely have a particular image. Whatever the
    sector – and you may well be involved with several – you are still
    relaying positive messages about yourself and your job through your
    overall image.

    the location
    The demands and attitudes of a cosmopolitan metropolis are certainly
    very different to a smaller provincial industrial town or, indeed, a rural
    market one.

    the weather and the season
    It is not just the practical aspect to be taken into account. Certain
    fabrics can look inappropriate as the texture and weight matter as much
    as colour.

    the corporate image
    If your company does have an image, make sure that you reflect it
    whilst also portraying your own individuality.

    your status
    Check that you look the level that you are ... or higher.

    The personal factors
    your age, *your* bodyshape, *your* personality, *your* lifestyle and *your*
    budget.

    your aspirations
    It is said that if you look the part of the next rung on the ladder, you
    will most likely be chosen for the role.

**Although it would be nice to spend unreservedly on our wardrobe, expensive clothes in
themselves are not the answer to a positive and successful business image.**

THE MISBELIEF

If you could spend a fortune on your clothes,
you would look a million dollars.

THE TRUTH

You may *feel* like a million dollars but it really ends there. You actually
would look no different than you do in your normal High Street togs . . . and
you would be a great deal poorer!

THE ANSWER

How to look a million dollars without actually spending it

Choose investment garments *with skill*

Ensure they fit and flatter

Co-ordinate and accessorise correctly

Compliment and Complement with Good Grooming

Let us first define what is generally accepted as Business Wear for the life you lead.

business wear for men

the suit

fabric

I would recommend that you always spend as much as you can comfortably afford but base your decision on fit, fabric, style, quality and cut rather than on a 'must-have' Designer name. The suit should always be of a medium weight fabric (350–400 grams) so that it hangs well. Cool wool is always the best alternative, possibly supplemented by a small proportion of man-made fibre to make it more crease-resistant and hardwearing. Do avoid synthetic fibres totally if you tend to perspire.

For warmer weather, the fabrics can be lighter weight (250–300 grams) but don't buy cotton or linen suits unless you want to look like a ragbag. It is only suave Italian fashion models and shop window dummies that seem to get away with making creases look desirable!

colour

Except for really warm weather or travel to better climes, you should preferably choose a darkish suit. However, that doesn't mean you should limit yourself to a wardrobe of plain grey and navy. When the time comes for shopping, do look around as there are many acceptable colour variations. There are *low-key* checks or stripes that add interest and many degrees of greys, blues and brown hues – even very subtle greens. Do try black – but trust your eye. If you think you look like an undertaker or a headwaiter, leave well alone! However, a black mixture with a stripe, subtle check or texture may well be the compromise and an interesting addition to the closet. On the other hand, men often choose a garment solely on the basis that it looks 'different' but they do not bother to judge whether it is *suitably* different.

> **Subtlety and sobriety** in colour, shape or texture
> does not *have to* mean
> **dull or boring**

The only time to wear a lighter coloured suit is in spring, summer, or very early autumn when a paler grey, a French (lighter) navy, taupe, camel or Houndstooth check can look very good. But be aware of the limited practicalities – and to always finish your outfit with the right shoes.

style

As it takes some time before styles radically change, there are certain elements that will help you check that you do not look really out-of-date:

- Lapel width

- Jacket length and shape

- Buttoning style – single or double, number and how high

- Trouser width and shape (full, flared or straight), pleats and turn-ups (a single or double pleat is very much more flattering and comfortable for the not so slim).

- Pocket style – inset or flaps

- Back vents – single, double or none at all

TIP

Many men find their trousers go very shiny. It is useful to buy two pairs of matching trousers and rotate them. In any event, you really should not wear the same suit two days running.

smart/casual

In certain areas there is a definite or an implied *Dress Down* policy. I believe strongly that this should always still be Business Appropriate and based on what we call Smart Casual. This dress code has given rise to a great deal of angst among us Brits to whom these words are often a total enigma. However it really is very easy once you know how! It is usually a more European look that is based on well-chosen and matched co-ordinates rather than on the business suit.

If you have noticed the acceptability of this within your own business life, or if you often travel abroad for work, consider a jacket or two to wear with co-ordinating trousers. You can wear it with a tie or not as the case may be.

choosing the jacket

a blazer

Can be single or double breasted but the classic blazer that you have owned for a few years, possibly sporting brass buttons, can look very passé now and probably is a tad too short.

a "sports jacket"

Can be either single or double-breasted. It also could be either tailored, or rather more unstructured for less formality.

a blouson – suede or leather

This can look really good if worn correctly but will undoubtedly make for a rather less smart outfit than either of the other two options. An over abundance of zips or other trimmings may also detract from the fact you mean serious business.

colour

Classic colours are navy and black but dark shades like bottle or olive green, burgundy, caramel, etc. are a little more interesting whilst still perfectly acceptable. If appropriate to your personality, job and status, aqua, mid-blue and rust are rather more adventurous. All will look fine but again *only* if twinned with dark trousers for most formality; and chinos, cords or tailored jeans for least.

patterns and textures

You could now be a little more daring with tweeds, mixtures, and checks as long as they produce an overall look that is subtle.

choosing the trousers

The trousers should be tailored like suit trousers, of wool or wool mixture and in a dark colour for the maximum business-like look. Cords and chinos – tailored like trousers but not like jeans – add further informality whilst denim/moleskin etc. jean styles go even further towards a casual image.

Lighter shades and weights only become appropriate in warmer weather and should always look compatible with the jacket.

e.g. winter "brushed" cotton in a darkish colour looks fine with winter tweed whilst summer weight or light-coloured cotton would not.

There is a wide range of Smart/Casual as shown in the table below.

A smart tailored jacket coupled with dark trousers is really only one degree less formal than a suit.

degrees of smart/casual formality

Most formal   **co-ordinated with dark tailored trousers**

A blazer with a white/cream/pastel shirt and tie

A Sports jacket with a white/cream/pastel shirt and tie

A blazer or Sports jacket with a co-ordinating casual shirt and no tie*

A blazer or Sports jacket with a crew or polo neck*

A blazer or Sports jacket with a t shirt*

A leather or suede jacket or other blouson with a co-ordinating casual shirt and no tie*

A leather or suede jacket or other blouson with a crew or polo neck*

Less formal   **A leather or suede jacket or other blouson with a T-shirt***

* will look even more informal when paired with tailored cords, chinos or smart jeans

For those who feel comfortable wearing it, a further option is to wear an appropriate suit of a fashionable style with a black or white crew, t-shirt or sweater.

business wear for women

Your clothes should always be chosen in a medium weight fabric so that they hang well.

It is best to go for darkish shades but don't limit yourself to a wardrobe of plain grey and navy. When the time comes for shopping, look around as there are many acceptable variations on standard colours. Try rose, burgundy, olive, khaki, bottle, French navy, air force blue, teal, charcoal, taupe, terracotta, cinnamon, toffee, etc. Also consider low-key checks, stripes, tweeds and woven textures that add further interest. Avoid details like novelty buttons, appliqués, fringing at all costs both in terms of appropriateness and of shelf life.

For the sake of propriety, business wear should always include a jacket of some sort.

jackets

The suit or jacket should be simply elegant, tailored to some degree and not quirky or extreme. Never be too sexy – i.e. tight, short or revealing – but that does not mean that it cannot be fitted or shapely.

In terms of formality, the order could be considered:

1   A skirt suit*or a jacket with matching dress

2   A trouser suit*

3   A dress with a co-ordinated jacket

4   A Knitted 2 or 3 piece

5   Jacket and co-ordinating skirt or trousers*

* Dressed up or down by the use of accessories and tops

skirts

Straight skirts are the most elegant for all shapes and sizes – providing they fit well. Even if your hips are rather bigger than the rest of you, a straight skirt is the only universally flattering modern shape.

Length should currently be somewhere between just above the knee to just covering it. If you really will only wear a long skirt, it should be very long but still showing some leg above the ankle.

trousers

For business purposes, wear only tailored trousers in a cool wool type fabric/mixture with a narrow to medium-wide straight leg – and most definitely not leggings, cut-offs, drainpipes, Capris or jeans.

tops

Keep tops simple too – and not too skimpy! V or round necks sit best under most jackets as they create a flattering frame to the face. Lowish necks are not suitable for office wear as they may send out the wrong messages . . . and distract. In any case, when worn under a jacket they are usually not as flattering to either the jacket or the wearer.

To adapt to Smart Casual, you can include smart cardigans worn instead of a jacket and sweaters instead of blouses or tops.

Now that we have defined what is generally appropriate for both men and women, you must sort out in your own mind what is right for you and your job to create *your* Wardrobe that Works for Work.

summary

Business wear must always be

> **immaculate**
>
> **contemporary**
>
> **stylish**

Appropriate to:

the sector	**location**
weather	**the corporate image**
your status	**personal factors**
your aspirations	

Whatever the outfit, whether a suit or co-ordinates, the Finishing Touch is *most* important

> **good grooming**
>
> **appropriate accessorising**
>
> **clever co-ordinating**
>
> **flattering fit**

It will make all the difference

notes

creating your wardrobe that works

Everyone needs *their* wardrobe to work. You can then get on with the important things in life in the knowledge that you always know what to wear and *how* to wear it.

For working men and women this is even more imperative.

Now that we have established what is appropriate for your Business Image, you need to check out your own wardrobe and then decide what needs to be adjusted or added.

It should contain:

- An easily extracted capsule wardrobe so that packing is no longer a chore.
- 100% that you wear – no more mistakes.
- Something for every occasion – no need to panic buy.
- Items that reflect your selected self-image.
- Comfortable, practical and flattering garments that are 100% right for you.
- Less which is more – proper planning optimises the permutations.
- Clothes that earn their keep – crossover from day to evening; work to play.

To build your Work Wardrobe that Works effectively, it needs to work just for you and you alone. There is no magic formula that suits all; certainly not if it is going to do the best it can *for you*. For it to work as well as we would like it to, it should be considered a philosophy based on certain personal criteria:

1. you

your	Physicals
	Budget
	Personality
	Chosen Image
	Lifestyle

2. wardrobe management

Edit

Audit

Plan

3. the finishing touch

Appropriate Accessorising

Clever Co-ordinating

Flattering Fit

4. intelligent shopping

the work wardrobe that works

1. you

- **your physicals**

The characteristics, shape and proportion rather than the actual size.

- **your seasonal budget**

Be realistic – to keep it updated, you will need to regularly add to your wardrobe for it to work.

- **your personality**

You must wear the clothes, they must not wear you.

- **your chosen image**

This is already established – a successful business (wo)man!

- **your lifestyle**

In Table 7, roughly assess the percentage of your time spent on each activity you engage in and the number of different outfits that you would need for each in a month.

Then break it down further into Smart and Smart Casual, and then Daywear and Evening.

table 7

% time spent	activity	total outfits needed	total smart/ casual		total smart	
			day	eve	day	eve
	work – conferences etc					
	work – normal					
	work related – social					
	private social					
	sport/ physical recreation					
	interests and leisure					
	holidays					
	children (School transport, activities)					
	other: e.g. voluntary work etc.					
	MONTHLY TOTAL					

2. wardrobe management – edit

We shall now examine and sort your present working wardrobe.

- Remove everything that is not relevant to the current season – i.e. winter or summer.

- Put items at one end that only could be used a) for evening and b) for special occasions.

- The really casual that do not have a place in the working wardrobe should be put at the other end.

- You now should only be left with mainstream daywear.

- **For men**: Separate the suits, jackets, trousers and shirts into sections and put on uniform hangers.
  For women: Separate all your suits, trouser suits, dress and jackets etc. into *individual* items and then hang in sections and on uniform appropriate hangers – jackets, trousers, skirts, dresses, shirts/blouses/ tops.

A Word on Hangers:

Please do throw away all those horrid wire hangers from the Dry Cleaners. Invest now for life in some really good ones that allow you to see exactly what you have and keep your clothes in good shape. You will also get a great feeling of satisfaction if all your hangers match and clothes are hung the same way round. However nice the padded and the solid wooden ones look, they do take up seriously more space. I would therefore recommend the non-slip plastic ones that are much slimmer and hold the garments on firmly. For skirts and trousers, the best answers are peg hangers or those with expanding waists.

now...

You should be able to see clearly what you have.

You must be very honest with yourself.

- Set aside items that need attention – if you have not dealt with them within two weeks, eliminate them as you probably never will!

- The time has come to jettison *anything* that you know is inappropriate, dated, shabby, unflattering, uncomfortable or doesn't fit – and is unlikely to do so in the foreseeable future.

Now discard anything that does not feel and look 100%.

If this involves several garments, do not panic.

You probably have not been wearing them anyway!

> Most of us tend to want to keep our clothes for posterity.
>
> The trouble is that your shape, and the *fashion* shape, undoubtedly change over time.
>
> Even if something doesn't appear old fashioned, what may have fitted – and flattered – a few years ago, most certainly may not now.
>
> **Look at each item with your eyes – not foremost with your pocket or your heart!**

If you do this properly, the selection may appear considerably reduced. This will particularly apply if you are a hoarder, have not paid much attention to the wardrobe for quite a while or not recognised its importance to your Business Image.

However, the reality is you will actually be wearing all the same clothes that you have been, but now you just will be able to see them clearly, work out more combinations and plan what is needed to extend their use.

Once you have de-toxed the main wardrobe, do the same with all your accessories.

2. wardrobe management – audit

- List what you have left in categories on Table 8.

Suits	Skirts*
Jackets	Coats and outdoor jackets
Shirts (tops etc*)	Dresses*
Trousers	Knitwear

  * women

- Create outfits and list each outfit below on Table 9 with complementary accessories, adding more rows if needed. If your outfit is a complete item – like a suit or dress – just enter straight across the columns.
- Classify each as **SC (Smart Casual)** or **S (Smart)**.

table 8 – wardrobe audit

All suitable items from the current wardrobe

	winter	summer
jackets		
trousers		
shirts blouses (f) tops (f)		
ties (m) skirts (f)		
dresses		
outerwear		
knitwear		
shoes belts bags		
other		

what you need to buy

	winter	summer
jackets		
trousers		
shirts blouses (f) tops (f)		
ties (m) skirts (f)		
dresses		
outerwear		
knitwear		
shoes belts bags		
other		

table 9

men

jacket	trousers	shirt	belt

shoes	other	sweater	SC/S	outfit no
				1
				2
				3
				4
				5
				6
				7
				8
				9
				10

women			
top layer	**bottom layer**	**in-between layer**	**bag**

If you haven't got the *right* pieces to make a complete outfit, it cannot be considered an outfit. Should this be the case, you must judge whether it warrants buying what it needs in order to make it complete. If it would, ensure that the new addition can also be used to create further combinations.

shoes	other accessory	day/ evening	sc/s	outfit no
				1
				2
				3
				4
				5
				6
				7
				8
				9
				10

2. wardrobe management – plan

don't be *too* specific

WRONG
I need another lemon shirt (or top)* to go with my grey suit because my old lemon shirt (or top)* is shabby

RIGHT
I need a new shirt to go with my grey suit so I will buy one that complements the suit and that looks and feels good on me.

* women

Check if your total number of outfits answers all your requirements in relation to Table 7. If-not, list what you need to buy on Table 10 in order to expand what you have already.

checklist

* A raincoat, coat or outdoor jacket? It should be large enough to sit well over your jackets.

* More suits.

* A jacket or blazer. If you have one, possibly add the other.

* Trousers – Work out what colours and fabrics they should be by checking:

     What you want them to match that you already have or are going to buy?

     Should they be tailored or casual?

     Have you the all the basic colours – black, grey, navy and dark brown?

* Shirts (tops*) that will provide more combinations or update existing outfits *providing they are worth spending further money on.*

* Knitwear is a good device to adapt smart to smart-casual. Polo and crewnecks in basic colours like cream, black and navy are evergreens.

Men: Ties are your individuality label. But would a new one really breathe new life into an old suit?

Women: Perhaps a dress in a core colour would be useful to be dressed up or down as needs be.

table 10	
what you need to buy	
item	**to create an outfit with**
1.	
2.	
3.	
4.	
5.	
6.	
7.	
8.	
9.	
10.	

3. the finishing touch – appropriate accessorising

the etceteras

Umbrellas, glasses, your pen, wallet, folder etc may all be noticed by others so be sure they are worthy of you. However, I would like to stress that does not mean an over abundance of visible Designer logos.

men

shirts

For shirts that will be worn with ties, always wear cotton or cotton mixed with a small amount of polyester. Always check that the collar is ironed well, not showing any wrinkles or any fray at the points. For choice, you can't beat white and cream but *very pale* grey, lemon, pale blue, mid-blue and pink are all generally acceptable. I would recommend you to steer clear of the fashion items like checks, black, dark grey and all the deep shades unless fashion plays a big part in your life – and your career.

Cut away collars are the most popular, button-downs are usually considered more casual and tab collars hold the tie very tight giving a sharp point and a very Continental look.

Cuffs can be single or double and should extend beyond the jacket sleeve for smartness – about one quarter to one half an inch depending on your shape and height.

Although it is the current trend for appearing "Cool", (not in temperature, but in style!), wearing your normal suit shirt without a tie will never look *very* casual but, if you do, remember to always leave the top button undone. For shirts chosen to wear without ties, you can choose a much greater variety of colours, textures and fabrics. In fact, one could almost say that for winter fabrics, the heavier the appearance of the fabric, the more casual you will look. And the converse in Summer.

In my opinion, although one that I know to be controversial (even with my own sons!) short sleeved shirts can never look elegant – under any circumstances. Far better to wear a well fitting, not too tight, long sleeved one with the cuffs undone and tidily rolled back to midway between wrist and elbow.

ties

Why would any man think his tie should be "a bit of a laugh"? Please, please, don't make your tie – or yourself – a joke by choosing one with cartoon characters, slogans etc.

Subtlety is the key. Don't let your tie be what is remembered about you. The best ties are ones that co-ordinate to your suits and possibly include some small amount of the colour of the shirt.

The favourite knot at present is the Half Windsor which sits best under the cut-away collar.

belts

Basic black leather – plus tan, oxblood or dark brown if you have the shoes – are all that you really need.

braces

Better kept invisible.

shoes

Buy the best you can afford. Although you don't need masses, you really must not wear the same pair two days running. Shoes should always be clean, well fitting, comfortable and not scuffed.

Every man needs black shoes:

- Well structured like an Oxford Brogue or Derby *for suits and more formal jacket/trouser combinations*
- A casual lace-up or slip-on *for Smart / Casual*
- A soft shoe like a moccasin or loafer *for very casual*

Tan or oxblood can be worn selectively with other outfits such as a navy jacket and grey trousers – but always complemented by a matching belt.

Do remember that by wearing shoes lighter than your trousers, you are making your leg look shorter and drawing attention to your feet. An unbroken colour line is always the neatest and most preferable.

briefcase

Only leather and not *too* shabby. And pleeeease, do not carry holdalls, sports bags or the like as your workbag.

jewellery

Cufflinks etc should reflect your personality and the occasion.

A watch should also be sensible, manly and elegant, not humorous or childish brightly coloured plastic.

women

Jewellery, scarves and belts can add interest when the overall effect is too one-dimensional. But do not wear accessories just for the sake of wearing them.

jewellery

These should be subtle touches to customise and feminise your clothes.

Gold, silver, pearl, bronze and pewter are always right.

Not so small to be unnoticeable nor too big to overwhelm.

A small chain or similar round neck or a brooch finishes a simple well-cut suit.

shoes

Buy the best you can afford and remember that you don't need masses. Basic core colours to build your Wardrobe that Works i.e. Black, dark brown or navy – taupe or tan in warmer weather. Have different styles and heels for different purposes but you can never go wrong with simple stylish Courts that are not too clumpy-or too "mumsy".

Always protect with Scotchguard and re-apply regularly.

Shoes should always be clean, well fitting, comfortable and not scuffed.

bags

As for handbags, go for the best you can afford but restrict yourself to basic items in standard colours that will stand the test of time. One does not need a whole wardrobe of handbags today – often a large squashy bag and small evening bag can suffice. Although fashion has been advocating every colour bag with as much augmentation as possible, do remember that it is just a fashion and not really the right image for a businesswoman unless you need to convey an empathy with fashion itself.

For meetings and the like, it is always best to confine yourself to carrying one bag; If you need to accommodate a laptop, files etc., choose a feminine soft leather briefcase that will also accommodate all your personal items in a small inner bag.

hosiery

Sheer looking hosiery is fashionable but *Vaguely* or *Nearly Black* looks fine worn with most dark colours. Thick textured or opaque tights should be restricted to very short or long skirts and chunky shoes, not to be worn with business suits.

lingerie

Be measured expertly regularly (the boobs change every few years) to ensure you are buying the right size; it can make the world of difference to both comfort and appearance. Do not shun Panty girdles and Control tights which are definitely preferable to visible bulges.

3. the finishing touch – clever coordinating

- Clever co-ordinating is keeping co-ordinating simple. When creating an outfit, always work out which accessories you will add to complete it.

- Clever co-ordinating takes into account fabric and texture compatibility as well as colour.

- When combining separates of different colours, one item should contain some of the colour of the other by pattern, texture or trim. If it doesn't, you can create the link with your shoes – and belts, if you wear them.

- Clever co-ordinating depends on balance – the right length and width of garments must be judged by:

  your bodyshape

  your proportion

  the combination of the garments themselves

clever co-ordinating	
layer	
bottom	**top**
dress (any colour)	**jacket** (same colour as dress with different yet compatible texture)
	jacket (pattern which includes accessory colour + dress colour)
	jacket (accessory colour)
skirt (accessory colour)	**jacket** (accessory colour with different yet compatible texture)
	jacket (suitable contrasting colour)
	jacket (pattern to include accessory colour)
skirt (pattern to include accessory colour)	**jacket** (accessory colour)
skirt (contrasting colour)	**jacket** (accessory colour)
skirt (any colour)	**jacket** (any complementary colour)
suit (any colour)	

middle

| n/a |

| Contrasting colour |
| Small amount of light* + accessory colour |
| Light* |

| Accessory colour |
| Light* |
| Pattern linking colours in both skirt & jacket (+ minimum amount of light*) |

| A colour from the jacket pattern |
| Light* |
| Pattern to include accessory colour an compatible with jacket pattern |

| A colour from the skirt pattern |
| Light* |

| Same as skirt |
| Light* |
| Pattern in both skirt & jacket colours + small amount of light* |
| Pattern in either colour + small amount of light* |
| Accessory colour |

| Same colour but different texture |
| Light* |
| Pattern including suit colour (+/- accessory colour) |
| Pattern including suit colour + small amount of light* (+/- accessory colour) |

* Choose LIGHT as the shade that suits you and the garments best.
It could be brigth white, off white, cream buttermilk, ecru, ivory, milk etc.

women

- Keep to the basic colours – black, brown and navy. Remember that you don't need to wear brown clothes in order to have, and enjoy the benefit of, brown accessories. If you have the range of colours, choose which colour you will accessorise each outfit with by identifying:

  The most appropriate style for the circumstances

  The most flattering complement

- When combining separates of different colours, you can create the link with accessories by adding a scarf or obvious jewellery in the other colour, in a pattern of both colours or in your accessory colour e.g. jet, tortoiseshell or amber.

- In order to complete a total picture that works, you must always consider your accessories.

- By substituting a smart structured cardigan (not too fine) for a jacket, you can usually create a smart casual business outfit that is a tad less formal – but it does depend on the style.

- You can usually do the same with trousers as with skirts, depending on the shape.

- If accessory colour is black, you can usually perform the same co-ordinating with grey.

3. the finishing touch – flattering fit

Do not be afraid to alter your clothes but do ensure it is done professionally. However, if there were a great deal that needs to be changed, it would be best to find an alternative garment.

- The two lapels and both shoulders should line up.

- Trousers will only be comfortable if the rise coincides with yours.#

- Neither jackets nor trousers can ever hang as they should with overloaded pockets.

- There should not be any gape on buttons or pull on trouser pleats or seams which indicates tightness.

- There should not be extra material between the shoulder and the waist, usually visible in a crease at the neck.#

- The sleeves (or trouser legs) should not be cut too wide for your frame generally.

- The back of the neck sits properly tight to the nape of your neck.

- The armhole should not be too deep.#

- Your shoulders should be compatible with the shoulder seam.

- Sit down and move your arms around to ensure comfort.

#Alterations cannot usually alleviate this satisfactorily.

men

- Length of jacket must not be shorter than the middle knuckle on the thumb – and usually the length of the fully extended thumb when hands are hanging straight.

- Trouser hemlines should just reach the shoe and then break by folding slightly inwards. They should be long enough to conceal the first few laces of a laced-up shoe and be about one and a half inches longer at the back than the front.

women

- Bust should not be flattened.[#]

- The skirt should not be too wide at its base.

- Jackets should not finish just at your widest part – unless it's not too wide!

- Pockets and detail in the wrong place (e.g. bustline) draw attention to an area; they can often be moved or removed altogether.

Once you have considered all the outfits in the wardrobe in the light of the right co-ordinating and accessorising, all that now is left to do is to go shopping!

Intelligent shopping will make the most of your time, energy and budget whilst eliminating mistakes and impulse buys.

4. intelligent shopping

do's

- Use a back mirror to see your back view without turning.

- Wear socks/tights & shoes in the right colour and of the appropriate degree of smart or smart casual.

- Wear a top or bottom that will complement what you are selecting.

- Only focus on one need at a time.

- If matching an existing item, take it with or, at least, a button or cotton threads.

- Select to flatter your age, personality and bodyshape.

- Check for good fit and proportion.

- From time to time review your self ... nothing stays the same, especially us!

- Wear jewellery to dress up the potential purchase.*

- Wear make up and ensure that your hair looks presentable.*

don'ts

- Be a Fashion Victim or a Frump.

- Panic buy for a Special Occasion always look through your wardrobe carefully first and try and use something there.

- Play safe with duplicates of what you already have – or then go to the other extreme.

- Buy just because you don't want to go home without something.

- Stand on top of mirror – but at least 2 ft away.

- Ask others for advice unless you respect their appearance.

- Buy all one label, just for convenience, or you will look like their brochure.

- Buy 'MUST HAVES':

    "Seen it on someone/in a mag/in a shop window".

    "It's such a beautiful colour/fabric/pattern".

    "It's such a bargain".

    "Because a fashion pundit said so".

- Buy 'WHEN I AM' … thinner/tanned/have longer hair, etc.

You should be feeling very much more confident as we have examined all the elements of your presentation and your appearance. You now know what makes a positive business image and have applied it to yourself.

We are now at the point when we must make sure that your good work is maintained from now on and that you remember to review yourself from time to time.

Fortunately – or sometimes unfortunately – nothing stays the same!

summary

**You are well on your way
to *your*
Wardrobe that Works.**

you have
weeded the current wardrobe
dealt with those that need, and are worthy of attention
planned what you *need* to buy
learned how to put it all together
in order to
maximise the combinations
change the appearance
alter the functionality
and
always **look stylish**

notes

maintaing *your* wardrobe that works

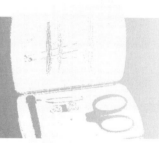

Now that you have a wardrobe that really works for you, *you* will also have to work for the wardrobe to ensure that it stays up to scratch.

caring for your clothes

- Leave clothes to air in the room overnight; check for threads, stains etc. and only put them away *when* they have been dealt with.

- Elastic waists should be hung on peg hangers to prevent the elastic stretching.

- Knitwear is best on padded or non-slip hangers to avoid it losing its shape.

- To keep them dust free, cover little-worn items with plastic shoulder covers.

- Always do up at least the top button of a garment to keep the shape and also pull out sleeves.

- To keep their shape, pad out handbags with rags, old towels or tissue.

footwear

- Always spray shoes with a protector before use *and re-apply regularly.*

- Check soles and heels regularly. Scuffed heels can be camouflaged with felt tip or a proprietary heel product.

- Never wear the same shoes two days consecutively.

- Always keep shoetrees in shoes. The best way is to invest in one pair of wooden trees (expensive!) and use them every night in the pair you have worn that day. They absorb perspiration and make sure the shoes last longer and keep their shape. The next day, substitute ordinary, cheaper plastic trees and vacate the wooden ones to be used over again.

- Suede should be regularly brushed with a special brush, using steam to remove stubborn stains and when faded, can be revitalised with Dasco spray in the appropriate colour.

- Patent is best cleaned with diluted washing up liquid and dried well with a soft cloth.

- When you lose one sock, use the other for polishing your shoes.

- Faded or dingy lingerie can be saved and then dyed all together in tea or in a snazzy colour.

- Use old pillowcases or acid-free tissue paper to pack clothes away instead of polythene which can discolour some fabrics.

- Avoid shine by always using a damp cloth when pressing clothes.

ties

- Untie the knot carefully after each wearing because leaving it knotted may cause permanent wrinkles.

- Always separate your ties into colour groups (e.g. those containing some navy, some grey, some black, etc) using either a wooden tie rack, a rail or hanger.

- Never trap your tie under your car seat belt which can cause silk to crease.

- Leave a few days in-between wearing a silk tie and hang it in a warm, moist environment to allow the creases to drop out.

- Never wash or rub a silk tie and preserve by using a silk protector.

Business trips can often put extra strain on the wardrobe. It is difficult to still look and feel your best living out of a suitcase without the facilities one has at home – or should have! The hints below may help you to maintain your image at home and abroad.

packing your clothes

- Roll all knits – they will be fine.

- Totally cover garments that tend to crease (cotton, linen, etc) with polythene covers which will minimise the creasing.

- Packing clothes on hangers saves time on arrival.

- Keep the shape of handbags and hats by filling them with underwear and other soft items.

- Always wrap cosmetics, toiletries and perfume in plastic or put in a separate bag within the case.

- It is often easier to take a smaller suitcase and a separate holdall for your shoes, bags, toiletries, etc.

- Use the sides of the case for shoes, books, belts, etc.

- Put the items on top that you are most likely to need first, e.g. a clean shirt, in case of delays.

- Always wrap shoes in case they are dirty.

- If time is of the essence, hang a complete outfit including the accessories on one hanger and cover totally with polythene.

- If anything does crease, hang in the bathroom immediately on arrival and let all the hot taps run **with the door closed** – the steam should do the trick. Hairdryers also work to blow out the creases.

The Wardrobe that Works could quickly become the wardrobe that *no longer* works. It has to be organised properly, and remain that way too, otherwise you could revert to old habits.

organising the wardrobe

hanging garments

- To maximise space, divide your cupboard into full hanging and half hanging.

- Trousers should be hung full length from extending waist or peg hangers.

- To get more out of full length hanging space, use 12" of chain around the neck of a hanger and insert the hook of another hanger through it.

- Use bars of soap tied with long ribbon, empty perfume bottles or pomanders to keep clothes smelling fragrant.

- Scarves, ties, belts and necklaces can be hung on hooks or a bar on the back of a cupboard door.

- Only ever hang one garment on each hanger.

- Use uniform hangers for the same type of garments. It is then much easier to find what you are looking for.

- Hang all similar items together e.g. trousers, skirts, jackets etc.

- Put all clothes *that can only be used for evening* at one end or in a separate wardrobe.

- Supermoths love natural fabrics. Ensure you use prevention; there is no cure except for costly invisible mending.

- Hang shirts rather than folding, even for packing, to minimise creasing.

Handbags should be kept in soft fabric bags or boxes identified by labelling or photos on the outside.

Shoes should be graded by colour.

Underthings should be separated into plastic bags or containers; drawer dividers are invaluable (available from John Lewis).

Life just has a way of playing some nasty tricks – and usually at the worst time possible – so 'be prepared'.

survival

- Keep needles threaded with white and black cotton somewhere easily accessible.

- Keep all spare buttons, material that has been cut off when shortening, etc. in a little bag together; you never know when you might need them.

- A lead pencil releases sticky zips.

- Colourless nail varnish or hair spray will stop ladders running further.

- Use Selotape on dark clothes, particularly shoulders, to remove fluff or stray hairs.

- Shorten sleeves quickly by folding over and adding press-studs.

- Double-sided tape holds for 24 hours and is invaluable for emergency patching.

- Lingerie clips will hold your bra straps in place. Tape or pin scarves and throws to feel more secure – it won't show!

- Shabby, light-coloured shoes can be painted silver, gold, etc. for evening.

- Woolite for silk, wool, cotton and linen can often be used when labels say 'dry cleaning only' and is more effective on certain stains.

- Cashmere Clinic for moth-nibbled garments: 020 7584 9806.

- Invisible mender: 020 7373 0514, 020 7487 4292, 020 7935 2487.

- Dyeing advice: www.dylon.co.uk.

- General advice: Good Housekeeping Institute at 020 7439 5000.

stains

Flush all stains immediately with soda water.

Blood   Soak in cold water with salt.

Grease   Soak stain in wash up liquid for 30 mins then wash as normal.

Pollen   Don't brush. Hold Selotape as near as you can without touching the fabric.

Chocolate Treat with glycerine and rinse in warm soapy water.

| Lipstick | Dab with eucalyptus and rinse in warm soapy water. |
| Perspiration | Dissolve Aspirin in warm water and soak. |

getting more from your wardrobe that works

for women

- Clip earrings can dress up court shoes or a bag for evening.

- A large scarf, or even a piece of fabric, worn under a jacket substitutes for a camisole or a blouse. But secure it well!

- Add a small piece of unobtrusive Velcro to a hat and re-trim it to match different outfits by adding buttons, bows, feathers, braid, etc.

- A small clutch bag can be converted temporarily into a shoulder bag (easier for drinks parties!) by adding a chain.

- Lighter-weight blouses and jackets can be re-vamped by cutting off the sleeves; similarly trousers can become abbreviated to shorts.

- Trim a simple dress or 2-piece with diamante or jet braid, buttons or fringing for a quick d-i-y cocktail outfit.

- Remove old-fashioned collars and convert to a granny neckline.

- Create a co-ordinated outfit by changing the buttons on a light coloured blouse to black and wear with a black skirt or trousers.

summary

**A positive image can only be maintained
when your wardrobe is maintained too**

By organising your wardrobe:

Items will be kept tidily in separate sections

You will see more potential combinations

Everything will be kept immaculate

Packing and unpacking will no longer be a chore

Despite best intentions, crises develop from time to time

Be prepared and there will be no need to panic at such times

notes

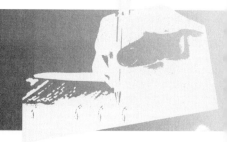

Now you know all about conveying a positive business image...

- **The ways in which you can use it.**

- **The components that make it up.**

- **The importance of monitoring other people's assessment.**

- **How to maximise all the Image Ingredients and make them congruent.**

It may take a little time for others to notice all the effects and for you to see their reactions. However, it really is best that way – your adjustments should be subtle and gradual, certainly not like the TV or magazine makeovers that are just short-lived fantasies.

Rome wasn't built in a day. Be patient and carry on with the good work and you most certainly will reap the benefits over time.

As we have agreed that nothing stays the same for long, there will always be some more work to do to maintain, or adjust, your positive image. However, now that you are enlightened, you can just take it all in your stride doing whatever is necessary quite naturally. Taking into account that you most certainly have learnt a great deal and are aware of the importance of keeping up a positive image, please do ensure that you set aside some time every few months to review yourself again. Armed with more confidence, you may well even take some new, and more adventurous, steps too.

Whenever there is any change in your life – a new job, location, promotion, season, etc, you will need to re-appraise. Obviously, this mainly applies to your clothes but all the other Ingredients should be considered too. For example, new situations may demand different etiquette or manners. However, with your new awareness, you will be able to make those judgements armed with the correct information and with added confidence.

checks

It would be so easy to sit back and be complacent now that you have done so much good work. We therefore need to prepare checks that can be carried out from time to time to ensure that the progress continues.

- Try the voice test with people who only 'meet' you on the phone.

- Deal with any mannerisms without becoming totally obsessed about them.

- Look in a mirror to see how you are walking and moving.

- Are you . . .

     . . . Sitting neatly?
     . . . Smiling as much as you can – and naturally?
     . . . Looking people straight in the eye when talking to them?
     . . . Not looking worried, tense or nervous?

- Is your grooming up to scratch?

- Ensure that your skin always looks clean, even, blemish free and healthy.

- If you wear glasses, check every so often that they still look modern.

- Keep your teeth white.

- Change your daily after shave or perfume sometimes.

- Make-up needs to be reviewed from time to time.

- The wardrobe most definitely needs to be reviewed each season and then dealt with accordingly. Requirements do change and you need occasionally to re-think in terms of the Wardrobe Management principles all over again.

It only remains now for me to wish you . . .

Good Luck

summary

You now know how to Manage *your* Image
In time, you will . . .

- make a positive First Impression
- raise others expectations of you
- achieve more positive outcomes
- be judged as confident
- make others confident in you too
- be viewed as successful
- feel more successful and begin to achieve more
- look good – and therefore feel good
- get more from people and situations
- ease your way up the ladder of success
- be viewed more positively by others
- communicate more effectively
- build relationships more quickly and easily
- be more visible, influential and credible

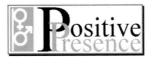

Dear Reader

At Positive Presence, our work is with men and women either as private individuals or within organisations.

We consult on every aspect of image and help people to get it right, or just "more right"! I do believe that for enhancement and development to work – and to be sustained – it has to be entirely appropriate to the person – to their personality, their lifestyle, status, budget, location, age and physical characteristics. But also to their aspirations.

Positive Presence is therefore different to other image consultants in that we do not work to a formula or a textbook; we judge every case individually, give guidance and help to make the changes accordingly. Because of this, it has been challenging to write a book that will be read and be useful to both men and women of all different ethnicity, ages, roles, locations and attitudes – and give advice that is relevant to all.

However the book has sold extremely well, been translated into Spanish and sold across five Continents – and with very positive reviews. I therefore feel confident that it offers a good basic guide for those whom we will never be able to help personally – or as an aide memoire for those we do.

Please do contact us if you would like to know more about Positive Presence for yourself, someone you know or for your organisation. We would welcome being advised of any opportunity where you think that I could be considered as a speaker, facilitator or presenter. This could be for your organisation, a social or networking group or at a particular event. I am regularly invited to address a wide variety of audiences both in the UK and abroad on a range of related topics and I would always be delighted to discuss possibilities with you.

Please do feel welcome to contact us with any questions, comments or to discuss any particular aspects of our work. We are now actively growing Positive Presence nationally and would really like to hear from you if you have a Positive Presence and are interested in becoming involved.

We look forward to hearing from you

Best regards

Laurel Herman

18a Lambolle Place London NW3 4PG
Tel: +44 (0)20 7586 7925   Fax: +44 (0)20 7586 7926
email: info@pospres.co.uk   www.positivepresence.com

Laurel Herman
speaker to business

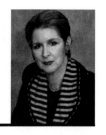

Laurel Herman is a leading international authority, innovator and thought-leader on overall personal development as well as being recognised as an expert in each of its relevant components – grooming, style and wardrobe, interpersonal communication, relationships, networking, etiquette and non-verbal behaviour.

Over the years Laurel Herman has enhanced the image, influence and impact of thousands of men and women and as Managing Director of Positive Presence, she also acts as a trusted personal adviser to several with a public profile and as mentor to rising 'stars'.

Laurel has written numerous articles for the trade and professional press as well as the definitive book on Business Image for the Chartered Management Institute which has been translated and sold across all continents. She frequently appears on TV, radio and in the press at home and abroad as a commentator and spokesperson. As Image columnist for CityAM, an expert for the Telegraph Business Clinic, a member of the Professional Speakers Association, the CIPD and the Association of Image Consultants International, she regularly presents to, facilitates for and addresses a wide range of audiences both in the UK and abroad.

Laurel is a sought-after accomplished and charismatic speaker recognised internationally for her expertise and knowledge. Over the years, she has spoken at numerous business events and gatherings both in the UK and abroad at which she is always well received. Because of her unparalleled hand-on experience making so many 'real' men and women more impactful, confident and successful, her stories and anecdotes make her a most inspiring and motivational speaker.

Currently very popular, her talk 'YOU are *your* own best Business Card©' (*when YOU walk in the door, it is YOU who wins – or loses – the deal, the job, or whatever else is at stake)* is an interesting, thought-provoking introduction to Impact Optimisation. Always customised to be relevant, it is informative whilst also giving some basic d-i-y tools for personal improvement.

As a successful entrepreneur, businesswoman and role model, Laurel is frequently invited to address women's networks and other Diversity related business audiences. Recognised as a seasoned graduate in Life and its challenges, an image doyenne who 'Walks her Talk' and an information resource, she also speaks on all aspects of appearance, confidence, being 'single again' and other issues of particular interest to women at Ladies lunches, pamper and lifestyle events.

about Positive Presence

the *intelligent* approach to image, impression and influence

When YOU walk in the door, it is YOU who wins or loses the deal, the job – or whatever else is at stake. It is no longer enough to be *just* competent, knowledgeable and professionally qualified. People buy people and as successful business is based on successful relationships, you need high personal impact to gain that all-important competitive edge.

Recognised as the *intelligent* image consultancy for *intelligent* people, Positive Presence is a leader in its field distinguished from others by its *intelligent* approach, reputation for excellence and exceptional client commitment.

To help organisations maximise their Impact Capital, Image Consultancy has been developed to a new groundbreaking level, Impact Optimisation. This unique three-faceted approach enhances and congruently integrates every aspect of how people look, sound and act in order to create a personal and professional Positive Presence. The exclusive Impact Optimisation programme, YOU are *your* own best Business Card©, provides the *intelligent* approach to image, impression and influence.

Laurel Herman founded Positive Presence in 1994 and, as an internationally acknowledged thoughtleader and authority in personal development, heads the team of hand-picked specialists in *every* aspect of personal and professional effectiveness. Their cumulative expertise, experience and perspective permits a wide range of consultancy and flexible interventions for organisations, teams and individuals on *any* particular aspect of impact and influence, whether relating to appearance, communication or behaviour.

the Positive Presence philosophy

For any development to be truly effective it must feel attainable, sustainable, affordable, authentic and personally relevant.

High Personal impact is directly linked to high levels of self-confidence, self-esteem and self-acceptance which are all underpinned by the Positive Presence Impact Optimisation process. Whilst never seeking to change people, this professionally brings out what is there *already* – and then works in partnership to make the *very* best of it. Our clients are then able to make informed adjustments which help them get the most from others, from situations … and from life.

the Positive Presence methodology

Using whatever communication style is appropriate, from logical and challenging to empathetic and sensitive....

... Dispels misconceptions and creates new thinking.

... Raises awareness about how others perceptions affect all interactions - and ultimately relationships.

... Motivates, inspires and empowers for contextual appropriate personal 'adjustment', not change.

... Delivers, harmonises and integrates a range of development and enhancement d-i-y tools and specialist interventions in every aspect of how we look, sound and act. (Appearance, Behaviour, Communication)

Positive Presence impact optimisation for INDIVIDUALS

Part 1 CONSULTATION *your* Personal Impact Factor

A confidential 2-hour session which can take place at Positive Presence premises or another suitable venue. It raises awareness, provokes new thought, dispels misconceptions, assesses the aspects for enhancement and development, defines attainable goals, motivates and inspires for appropriate change with some tools for d-i-y optimisation and maintenance.

optional

Part 2 OPTIMISATION – Others perception of you

Perception affects all interaction – and inevitably impacts on future relationships too. True impressions and perceptions are revealed by expertly extracting spontaneous feedback in two stages from a number of appropriate contacts nominated by the client.

Part 3 OPTIMISATION – Implementation

MODULES AND COURSES

APPEARANCE (A)	BEHAVIOUR (B)	COMMUNICATION (C)
'5-mins in the morning' make-up tutorial*	Cross-cultural awareness	Pitching with a Positive Presence
'Perfect shaving' tutorial*	Business or social etiquette	Effective writing
Hair makeover*	Working the Room with a Positive Presence	Interview techniques
Professional advice (e.g. Skin, Nails)	Raising your profile with a Positive Presence	Presenting with a Positive Presence
At-home Wardrobe audit	Networking naturally with a Positive Presence	Negotiating with a Positive Presence
Successful intelligent Shopping	Stress management	Positive Posture and movement
Wardrobe – personal styling	A Woman in a Man's world	Vocal presence and power
Business Appropriate	Confidence, De-clutter, Career, or Lifechange Counsel	Communicating with confidence & cred
Your Wardrobe that Works	Politics and Power in the workplace	Public speaking with a Positive Presence
De-mystifying Smart-Casual		Media skills
The Capsule Wardrobe		Effective Communication

all-inclusive personal plans

Discounted packages that include Parts 1, 2 and a pre-determined selection from A, B and C above.

Further details available on request.

what *they* say

Positive Presence is no ordinary image consultancy; it is an organisation that promotes an environment that changes people's lives. Laurel provides a wealth of talent and experience in spotting where there is the need for change, creative thinking – and the flair to ensure a positive outcome. The result has provided me with a platform and taken me to another level in appearance, attitude and confidence. The impact on the AAT is a President seen across the world who commands respect, holds attention, and who has led it into the 21st Century and is testimony of the work done by Laurel and her team. With their support and guidance, they have changed my life.

I therefore have no hesitation in unreservedly recommending Positive Presence to you or your organisation. They do "Change People's Lives".

Tim Light, President – ASSOCIATION OF ACCOUNTING TECHNICIANS

In our business, as in most, first impressions matter. The Positive Presence personal service has helped me to feel confident about appearing professional at all times and encouraged me to experiment in ways that I would not otherwise have explored.

I would recommend this service to anyone who wants to make their appearance business strength.

Peter King, Snr. Partner – SHEARMAN & STERLING LLP, London

Laurel is an outstanding intuitive coach who got to the heart of key issues that had been holding me back from both professional career advancement and in achieving important personal goals. I left the consultation not only with a clear vision of where I want to go but with the committed support by Laurel and her able team to help me get there.

I highly recommend Laurel and Positive Presence to anyone who is serious about making a positive impact.

Steven D'Souza, HR – MERRILL LYNCH

Laurel gave me invaluable advice on every aspect of my image as well as carrying out confidential feedback interviews with a number of my peers and more senior directors. She referred me to a number of her team, as well as taking my wardrobe in hand herself, and as a result I have changed my hair, my makeup and clothes as well as working on other areas of personal presentation. The changes in me have been positively noted from the Chairman of the Group downwards.

I believe they had a most significant part to play in a recent promotion (and pay rise!), together with the main board approval of my business plan for a (seriously expensive!) new venture.

Sarah Moynihan, Group Financial Controller – MARSHALL HOLDINGS (Cambridge)

I attended a workshop conducted by LH which was probably the best thing I have ever done during my career to date. Since meeting her, I have been able to address a number of issues very satisfactorily both personally and for my organisation. LH has an excellent way of making one at ease and tackle even most difficult matters either herself or via her very professional team. Laurel's style and advice is independent, objective and has helped me greatly to meet and progress all my career objectives.

I have no hesitation in recommending Positive Presence to anyone as this is a real asset to have.

Arif Kamal, Group Finance Director – G.L. HEARN

Positive Presence has worked with a number of my client teams and has supported Director and Partner candidates as they prepare for significant career milestones in all aspects of positive presence including voice, style, impact and clothes.

I am very pleased to report a 100% success rate to date.....

Robert Bryant, Partner – DELOITTE LLP

Positive Presence Impact Optimisation for GROUPS

This client-friendly and flexible programme can be delivered to teams or groups at any suitable venue in the UK or abroad but the greater the homogeneity of the group, the more effective the messages. Group options can be combined with one-to-one enhancement for key individuals and can be followed by ongoing team building and development.

The content always follows the same logical sequence with key messages that encapsulate the effective one-to-one development process but specific modules can also be included, substituted or stand-alone. The programme is available in several formats to facilitate meeting client requirements and to give best value. These range from an introductory 'taster' talk to a full length on-going course but also vary in style, emphasis and depth of detail. (see Delivery Variations).

contents

Part 1   Laying the Foundations

Your Image is their perception of you, not yours – examining the differences and the implications

Defining Personal Impact – it is ... and it is not...

Modelling Impact (aka credibility, gravitas, attitude, profile, polish)

Your Personal Impact factor (self evaluation)

Your Impact level is a decision made by others – when, why, how

Positive Presence is consistent Positive Impact + Positive Performance

Moving forward – making others make a positive impact decision about you

Managing the First Impression

Part 2   The Building Blocks

Making a positive First Impression within the context of first encounters selected from:

- Invisible Image – email
- Invisible Image – phone/teleconferencing – voicepower
- Meetings and video conferencing – appearance, voicepower, etiquette, body language
- Audiences – as above+media, presentation, public speaking, skills
- Business social – as above+initiating/developing/maintaining relationships, networking strategy and tools, personal profile raising and working the room

Addressing existing perceptions, situations and relationships that need improving.

DELIVERY VARIATIONS

EMPHASIS	A specific emphasis can be applied. e.g. *'How Americans see Brits'* and *'Women in a Man's World'*		
DEPTH OF DETAIL	Highly experienced, technically qualified members of the Positive Presence team of experts can be incorporated to deliver in-depth or advanced sessions in their specialism		
STYLE	Ranging from serious and instructional to light hearted edu-tainment		
FORMAT	TALK	1-2hrs	A 'taster' introduction to Impact Optimisation as a keynote and for breakout sessions at conferences, member events, team days, etc.
	ROUNDTABLE 'DISCUSSION'	1-2hrs	Fully interactive for Board members, very senior execs, etc.
	MASTERCLASS	1-3hrs	Partially interactive, for senior levels at accelerated pace
	SEMINAR	1-2hrs	Partially interactive tutorial
	WORKSHOP	*from* 2hrs	Fully interactive, can also include selected detailed modules presented by specialists from the Positive Presence team
	FULL COURSE	*from* 2dys	In-depth introduction + selected in-depth modules

MODULES and COURSES

Other related topics can be designed by the Positive Presence team of specialists on request

APPEARANCE (A)	BEHAVIOUR (B)	COMMUNICATION (C)
'5-mins in the morning' *make-up tutorial*	Cross-cultural awareness	Pitching *with a Positive Presence*
'Perfect shaving' tutorial	Business or social etiquette	Effective writing
Hair makeover	Working the Room *with a Positive Presence*	Interview techniques
Professional advice *(e.g. Skin, Nails)*	Raising your profile *with a Positive Presence*	Presenting *with a Positive Presence*
At-home Wardrobe audit	Networking naturally *with a Positive Presence*	Negotiating *with a Positive Presence*
Successful intelligent Shopping	Stress management	Positive Posture and movement
Wardrobe – personal styling	A Woman in a Man's world	Vocal presence and power
Business Appropriate	Confidence, Career, De-clutter or	Communicating with confidence & cred
Your Wardrobe that Works	Life change Counsel	Public speaking *with a Positive Presence*
De-mystifying Smart-Casual	Politics and Power in the workplace	Media skills
The Capsule Wardrobe		Effective Communication

what *they* say

Everybody that I spoke to found your talk very interesting and thought provoking and, without exception, took something useful away from it whatever level they were at in the organisation.
Andrew Hunt, Director   SMITH AND WILLIAMSON

In a very short amount of time Laurel was able to get across the importance of communication in all its forms and the fact that it does not matter how well you may be prepared on a technical basis, you only get one chance to make that first and lasting impression.
David Thomas,   Group Financial Director TDG LOGISTICS

I was most taken with your presentation and found the experience a good 'self-test'; it is often easy, when busy, to forget the need to make a good and positive 'first impression'.
David Wilson, Financial Director   PRICE FORBES (Participant – FD Forum)

I found Positive Presence to be extremely professional and keen to respond to my firm's specific needs. We have received excellent feedback from our staff and will definitely be working with Positive Presence again in future.
Amanda Dulieu, Director CREDIT SUISSE

Both my colleague and I found it thought-provoking, and, like the accompanying book, full of practical tips to help people gauge and improve their personal impact.
Juliet Brilliant, NETWORK RAIL (Participant – London Business School ALUMNI NETWORK)

The programme was a great success as a direct result of your commitment and efforts.
Clive Bannister, CEO HSBC

Your session made an excellent difference to all the others at the conference and was very well received by all who attended. Delegates particularly enjoyed hearing about the impact their image has on others. Thank you for such a wonderful presentation.
Doreen Baker, Audit Policy & Advice Team HM TREASURY

I thought that your presentation was intriguing and believe that it will prompt many of us to consider how we can improve personal effectiveness and impact through our own image and presentation.
Mark Allatt, National Business Development Partner DELOITTE LLP

I have heard nothing but compliment from all who attended the luncheon – and they are a very discerning audience.
Peter Chrome, General Manager CHEWTON GLEN

The response to your session was overwhelmingly positive. We are most grateful for your thorough and informative session and we will undoubtedly invite you again.
Philana Quick, Asst CLO US EMBASSY

Laurel is a wonderful speaker as she makes her audience feel so positive and enthusiastic about themselves and their lives and what they can achieve.
Fiona Wilson, Head of Family Law BLAKE LAPTHORN TARLO LYONS

An excellent event .... Laurel showed a natural empathy with her audience and had a style of presenting that was fully inclusive to all participants whether they be introverts or extroverts. A very valuable session with lots of practical tips.
Debs Eden, (Executive PA Magazine **PA of the Year) PwC**

The feedback from participants attending your workshop has been overwhelmingly positive. They found it engaging, energizing and inspiring. Thank you for being so kind as to offer a second, impromptu session due to the high demand of those who wanted to attend.
Marie O'Hara, Manager, External Relations W.I.N. (Women's International Networking) **CONFERENCE, OSLO**

Positive Presence for Organisations

The First (and lasting) Impression of your organisation
particularly for SMEs & Professional Service providers

When it comes to people, the importance of the First Impression and the effects of their image are universally recognised. Positive Presence is renowned internationally for its unique and successful approach to optimising personal impact of men an women in the workplace.

Similarly, the image value of an organisation significantly affects people's expectations – and future outcomes. Whereas insiders may know the reasons for certain negative aspects, others do not – and they draw their conclusions from *everything* that they see or hear. Many SMEs and professional service firms have grown organically without some key aspects of their overall business image ever being considered.

Image is the most important tool of communication and the face of a business should reflect its core values. The company and its people, both collectively and independently, should be perceived as attractive, successful and professional whilst always appropriate to location, sector and status. An overall positive image will give the organisation a cutting edge in the market place and encourage sales, investment, recruitment and employee retention.

Today, people buy people, not just products or services. When people achieve a positive image and attitude, their performance is enhanced and they undoubtedly become more confident, communicate better and more easily initiate and develop relationships. Together with the physical surroundings, they should reflect excellence which is easily attainable and sustainable once the appropriate tools and training are in place.

Positive Presence provides an objective and professional audit of everything that is seen and heard. We then create strategy to optimise your Impact Capital whilst meeting your budget and logistic constraints.

Typical areas to be considered may be:

- Telephone skills
- Internal and external décor & signage
- Rest rooms, meeting rooms and boardrooms
- Every channel of communication – Website, advertising, marketing & PR
- Hospitality – catering, concierge etc.
- The people within from the tea lady to the MD

- Literature and stationery
- Meeting and greeting
- External appearances at conferences, exhibitions etc.
- Reception areas and receptionists
- All equipment
- Transport vehicles

The process begins with the establishment of objective, budget, time, people and logistical constraints followed by a fact-finding exercise and assessment of the current situation. A summary and outline proposal is submitted after which a process and action plan are agreed. The optimisation programme is delivered with effectiveness measured and monitored by periodic reviews and top-up sessions.

Positive Presence clients span all sectors and all types of organisations from global corporations and Professional Bodies to SMEs, Partnerships and Sole traders.

Clients include...

GSK	HP	IBM	American Express	Shell	BP
Deloitte	PWC	KPMG	Ernst & Young	Credit Suisse	Citi
Clifford Chance	CMS Cameron McKenna LLP	Thomson Reuters	Bank of NY Mellon	Svenska Handelsbanken	Société Générale
HSBC	Eversheds LLP	DLA Piper	Manches LLP	Shoosmiths	Reed Smith Richards Butler LLP
Mazars LLP	Saffery Champness	Smith & Williamson	Freshfields Bruckhaus Deringer LLP	Linklaters LLP	BUPA
TDG Logistics Ltd	HM Treasury	Department for Education and Science	Department of Health	GL Hearn	DTZ
Lawson Dodd PR	Beachcroft LLP	Addleshaw Goddard LLP	ASB Law	Morgan Stanley	London Chamber of Commerce
Chartered Management Institute	Association of Accounting Technicians	CIMA	ICAEW	Institute of Chartered Accountants Australia	Association of Chartered Certified Accountants
Provident Financial	London Business School	Portsmouth NHS Trust	Cancerkin	Rural Payments Agency	Institute of Directors
Knight Frank LLP	Carillion plc	Vizards Wyeth	The Law Society	Girls Day School Trust	RPC LLP
Secondary Heads Association	University of Westminster	University of Middlesex	Girton College Alumni	UBS	Britannia Building Society
McDermott Will & Emery	Thomas Eggar Solicitors LLP	Nabarro Nathanson LLP	BMI Healthcare	Pfizer	Royal Marsden Hospital
Accenture	Lansons Communications	Weber Shandwick	Institute of PR	Proctor & Gamble	Wilkinson's Stores
IIR Conferences Ltd	IDDAS	Ceridian Centrefile	CIPD	Holiday Extras	Garland Call Centres
Richmond Events	Chewton Glen	US Embassy	The Foreign Office	Swedish Chamber of Commerce	ITV
Avenance Ltd	Wentworth Golf Club	Sodexo Ltd	Cox Insurance Holdings	Iron Trades plc	Lloyds of London
Cliveden Club	Vineyard at Stockcross	RAC Club	Meeting Industries Association	Hilton Hotels	The Lanesborough
Savoy Hotel Group	Mosimann's Private Dining Club	Sure Deodorant	Kaplan Hawksmere Ltd	Catamaran Cruisers Ltd	DBM (Hungary)
Price Forbes	Evening Standard	Global Leadership Forum (Switzerland)	Infercom (Finland) Ltd	Al Hilal Group (Middle East)	NAWBO (USA)
English Tourism Council	Virgin Atlantic	Institute of Home Economics	Champneys	Barclays plc	Sanctuary Healthcare
Lloyds TSB	Marshalls of Cambridge	DVLA	Basel Trust	Grosvenor Estates	United Biscuits plc
Click Group Ltd	Institute of Internal Auditors	Barlow Lyde & Gilbert LLP	Dawsons LLP	Institute of PR	Merrill Lynch
CB Richard Ellis	NatWest Securities	Prudential	London Borough of Camden	Grayshott Spa	Business Link
Management Forum Conferences	BT	University of Southampton	Sun Life Insurance of Canada	Mckinsey & Co.	JP Morgan
Inst. of Chartered Secretaries &Administrators	Multiplex Construction Ltd	Caribbean Cruises Ltd	Digby Trout Ltd	Forum Holdings Ltd	Ealing NHS Trust